ILLNESS and *Image*

ILLNESS and *Image*

Case Studies in the Medical Humanities

Sander L. Gilman

Routledge
Taylor & Francis Group
LONDON AND NEW YORK

First published 2015 by Transaction Publishers

Published 2017 by Routledge
2 Park Square, Milton Park, Abingdon, Oxon OX14 4RN
711 Third Avenue, New York, NY 10017, USA

First issued in paperback 2018

Routledge is an imprint of the Taylor & Francis Group, an informa business

Library of Congress Catalog Number: 2014010796

Library of Congress Cataloging-in-Publication Data

Gilman, Sander L., author.
Illness and image : case studies in the medical humanities / Sander L. Gilman, Emory University.
p. ; cm.
Includes bibliographical references and index.
ISBN 978-1-4128-5493-1 (alk. paper)
1. Human body--Social aspects--Case studies. 2. Body image--Psychological aspects--Case studies. I. Title.
[DNLM: 1. Human Body. 2. Body Image--psychology. 3. Culture. 4. Disease--ethnology. HM 636]
HM636.G55 2015
616.85'2--dc23

2014010796

ISBN 13: 978-1-138-51079-1 (pbk)
ISBN 13: 978-1-4128-5493-1 (hbk)

For Kai and Hana

Contents

List of Figures

Introduction

The Medical Humanities Today

The Medical Humanities and the Health Sciences

The medical humanities are (the plural is important) a nascent and evolving academic specialty, which are already an intrinsic part of higher education both for undergraduates in the health sciences, whatever their professional trajectory, as well as for professional students. In this volume the health sciences should be understood as not just human medicine but also fields such as nursing, public health, dentistry, disability studies, and all other fields that deal with human illness and wellness. I am excluding veterinary medicine here, but analogous questions exist in this field also. The field of the medical humanities stresses the value of traditional humanities and social science approaches to the widest range of questions and problems dealing with human health and illness. It also has a role in the education of health science professionals without denigrating the research and teaching undertaken at professional schools of medicine, nursing, dentistry, and public health.

Our contemporary sense of the medical humanities evolved in the 1960s in concert with the development of medical ethics, although they have subsequently evolved along different paths. Unlike medical ethics, which for a long time was the stepchild of academic philosophy, the medical humanities are not indebted to a single discipline. It may become a unified discipline over time, but what it is right now is a series of disciplinary methodologies (encompassing the plurality of approaches found within disciplines from art history to literary criticism to medical and social history to anthropology, sociology, etc.) as applied to an ever-growing range of questions and problems concerning the health sciences. These methodologies converge as they are applied to a Venn diagram of overlapping health science topics, from creating a professional medical identity to illness to health to patient definitions to hospital design to disability studies, to the very definitions of "health" and "science" within the health sciences.

The medical humanities are an acknowledgement that multiple perspectives can and do provide different and coherent approaches to complex and often contradictory questions beyond the traditional scope of the humanities. As part of the medical humanities, the arts, too, have developed a relationship with the health sciences. From literature to the widest spectrum of the visual and musical arts, the health sciences now serves both as the subject of such works (as has always been the case) but also as a means of better approaching and comprehending aspects of the health sciences. For instance, learning to "see" patients can be first approached by understanding what "learning to see" *is*, either in the context of the art museum or in the production of works of art. What is interesting is how these disciplinary approaches to such objects—no matter what their theoretical presuppositions—can, when juxtaposed, present a deeper understanding of the clinical and research agendas of the health sciences as well as humanities and "soft" social sciences. This mutual acknowledgement of common value is important in the medical humanities. Here is a moment when the now undervalued humanities can stand on its own, using its multiple methodologies and approaches in new and critical ways.

The medical humanities are neither ancillary to another field nor are they peripheral to the humanities in and of themselves. They may indeed come to be part of evidence-based practice or evidence-based medicine, as the definition of scientific medicine also has expanded to include new and innovative approaches.[1] The definition of scientific evidence also has expanded to include new and innovative approaches, evidence, and questions, as in the application of biosocial, cultural, and situational determinants to the study of diseases. Today one cannot hide behind a reductive claim that evidence-based medicine in its narrowest sense is real science and that the introduction of interpretation and history as advocated by the humanities therefore deflects from it. The philosopher Charles Taylor notes that a physician cannot simply declare: "I'm going into medicine because I can really do a lot of good and I know I can do a lot of good, because of the scientific grasp that I have and I just don't want to have to deal with these other deep issues, which I might if I had more confidence in myself, but I don't want to agonize over them."[2] For evidence-based medicine itself, from the time of Hippocrates, relies and relied on interpretation of "seeing" or, to use its technical term, diagnosis.

To see means to interrogate. The sole physician to sign the Declaration of Independence, the Philadelphia doctor Benjamin Rush (1746–1813) lectured his medical students that:

> Physicians by reviewing the history of complaints from their patients will often have them exaggerated but by frequent visits you cannot be deceived. . . . Endeavor to get the history of the disease from the patient himself and do not interrupt him till he has finished as he will always give the best symptoms tho' he may give the worst causes. Begin to interrogate your patient. By how long he has been sick? When attacked and in what manner? What are the probable causes, former habits and dress; likewise the diet, etc., for a week before especially in acute diseases. . . . In chronic diseases enquire their complaints far back and the habits of life. . . . Pay attention to the phraseology of your patients, for the same ideas are frequently conveyed in different words. A pain in the precordia is called by an Englishman a pain in his stomach, by a Scotchman in his breasts, an Irishman in his heart and by a Southern man mighty poorly. Enquire of your patients the diseases of their ancestors, the age to which they lived and the remedies which relieved them. It is of consequence because there is a hereditary idiosyncrasies in some families. Patients often conceal the cause of their disease—therefore interrogate them particularly when you suspect intemperance as the cause of disease.[3]

Knowing the approach by which you interpret what you see makes you a better diagnostician, and learning those theories of interpretation means studying the medical humanities as a physician in training or indeed as a potential patient. The context of diagnosis is closely tied to the health sciences' claims about prognosis—that is, you know the world in terms of your interpretation of the world. Hans-Georg Gadamer noted in *Truth and Method* that interpreters must be "sensitive to the text's alterity," which demands the rejection of any type of "neutrality" (such as the claims of objectivity) and an articulation of "the validity—of the fore-meanings dwelling within him." "The important thing is to be aware of one's own bias," Gadamer states, and that means understanding the context in which one interprets, even if one's understanding is fragmentary and incomplete.[4]

The medical humanities are valuable to the health sciences because they use evidence generated by the methodologies of the humanities to augment that evidence traditionally generated within the health sciences. When we look at all of the debates about and within the humanities concerning the health sciences, we can observe that these contradictions are not a problem of the humanities but a quality of the generation and transmission of knowledge within the greater scope of intellectual life. Thus the literary critic Andrew Delbanco argues that the humanities are inherently better than the health sciences. For "[T]he questions we face under the shadow of death are not new, and... no new technology will help us answer them."[5] Science's "principle of progress" does not "translate well" into other areas of human life: "Science tells us nothing about how to shape a life or how to face death.... It not only fails to answer such questions; it cannot ask them." Delbanco knows that some scientists have predicted that in time "neuroscience will define and ensure happiness and ... biochemistry will distinguish truth from falsity among what today are mere opinions about sex and gender," but he doubts "it will happen"; even if it does, "none of us will be around ... and it's not clear that we would want to be."[6] The fact is that the medical humanities already integrates all of these questions without denigrating the state of the science itself. And yet the reflection of the world of the health sciences in the teaching of the humanities has been marginal at best, both on the undergraduate and the graduate level.

What the medical humanities as a developing field now offer to students studying the health sciences or the humanities is a field of action in which complex problems and questions regarding the generation of knowledge come under the lens of methodologies that are not identical to the methodologies generating the knowledge itself. We see the world through multiple lenses: the medical humanities provide a series of such lenses. Charles Taylor noted that in the end we are all "self-interpreting animals," each of us constituted in part by an ongoing, and open-ended process of collective self-interpretation.[7] The health sciences are thus innately different from the natural sciences because the objects of the health sciences are us, "self-interpreting animals," and what constitutes our humanness, and that of the health sciences, is to no little degree the way that we are constantly reinterpreting who and how we are. This is especially true within clinical practice.[8] Jürgen Habermas has argued that this process of self-interpretation is not merely limited to questions of our performance of identity and our various roles in society, but rather incorporates questions regarding what it actually means to be human.[9] This book will enable us to see how some concepts like "hygiene" and "mental disorder" are a means by which human beings are able to constitute historically who they think they are. Such images are part of the vocabulary within which we think and describe our identities as human beings, whether we are health professionals, patients, observers, or all of the above.

Looking and Seeing (and Hearing)

We are constantly looking at the world. What we see is clearly determined not only by the complex mechanism of sight but by our processing of such impulses through our understanding of the way we see the world. This understanding alters with time. Thus in 1834 the English physician and physiologist Marshall Hall (1790–1857) could stress the centrality of the face in seeing the patient:

> The countenance of the patient, although a source of information too much neglected by writers on medicine, is very peculiar and highly characteristic in many diseases, and affords to the physician of experience and observation an important mean of diagnosis. The kind, the stage, the changes, the mitigation and the progress of many morbid affections are accompanied and denoted by corresponding states of the countenance. . . . It is impossible not to be impressed with the importance of changes in the countenance so observable, so diversified, and so characteristic, with a view to every practical purpose in the art of medicine.[10]

Hall's claim that this is a new approach may seem odd, as we know that physicians from the time of Hippocrates were recoding the visible symptoms and coordinating them into systems of diagnostic classification. Hall's view is new because he is focused on and fascinated by reflexes, the nervous system in its visual manifestation, and so begins to see the world, including forms of mental illness, as visible and observable. What he sees in looking at the faces of his patients is the unseeable but not unknowable world of the nervous system in action.

Even the introduction of technology, now so very pervasive in the health sciences, does not mediate our need for an understanding of how we learn to see and know the world. In 1761, Leopold Auenbrugger (1722–1809) introduced the physician to the sounds generated in the body by tapping on the thorax:

> I here present the reader with a new sign, which I have discovered for detecting diseases of the chest. This consists in percussion of the human thorax, whereby, according to the character of the particular sounds thence elicited, an opinion is formed of the internal state of that cavity. In making public my discoveries respecting this matter, I have been actuated neither by an itch for writing, nor a fondness for speculation, but by the desire of submitting to my brethren the fruits of seven years' observation and reflection.[11]

He had observed his father tapping on kegs of wine to judge their fullness. It was his ability to examine that which was unseen but now knowable that startled his contemporaries. Technologies—from stethoscopes to the fMRI—have not and will not make known all that is unseen but known about illness, as they are always a product of that world's understanding of health and illness that generated the technology.

Auenbrugger's act of knowing not just through seeing but also through hearing was taken up by René Laennec (1781–1826), who improved on it by introducing a new technology, the stethoscope. He speculated on how this type of mediation changed his way of knowing:

> In 1816 I was consulted by a young woman labouring under general symptoms of diseased heart, and in whose case percussion and the application of the hand were of little avail on account of the great degree of fatness. The other method just mentioned [direct auscultation] being rendered inadmissible by the age and sex of the patient, I happened to recollect a simple and well-known fact in acoustics, . . . the great distinctness with which we hear the scratch of a pin at one end of a piece of wood on applying our ear to the other. Immediately, on this suggestion, I rolled a quire of paper into a kind of cylinder and applied one end of it to the region of the heart and the other to my ear, and was not a little surprised and pleased to find that I could thereby perceive the action of the heart in a manner much more clear and distinct than I had ever been able to do by the immediate application of my ear.[12]

The subtleties of the approach are determined not only by what one hears, but how one hears it. The patient here generated the technology because of a combination of conventions about the role of gender within medicine (how does a male physician *modestly* listen to the beating heart of a young woman) as well as the knowledge of acoustics, physiology, and interpretation.

Seeing and Knowing as Central to the Medical Humanities

In this volume I shall be looking at how the medical humanities can use evidence from the health sciences and be in a critical dialogue with them about the meanings inherent in their problems and methods. Such a dialogue must take both sides of the equation, the humanistic and the medical, seriously without claiming any primacy. I shall examine the function of representations of the world in the health sciences through a series of case studies that rely on a critical reading of the science as part of a disciplinary structure as well as of the science as part of general culture. I shall be asking how such moments, seen historically as well as critically, provide us with some insights into the meanings that we all attach to images of health and illness. These meanings permeate both the assumptions in the humanities as well as in the health sciences.

In their critical paper on representations in the health sciences, Roger Cooter and Claudia Stein point out the limits of visualization and interpretation in the existing literature on the public representation of health and illness.[13] They focus on the complex and multilayered field of medical representations as the site where levels of epistemic, philosophical, and political presuppositions provide insight into the interpreter's historical position. From a close focus on medical (or even public health) representations as a reflection of a partial worldview to the historical embeddedness that Cooter and Stein suggest is the key to understanding the limitations of all visual hermeneutics in the sphere of health and illness:

> . . . historians seeking to use visual materials need to be aware that any instruction as to their use is a priori discourse laden. The coming into focus of health posters in the 1990s and visual culture in general as something of seemingly great importance, something for serious critical engagement, is but a perception of one particular socio-cultural moment (precisely that which we have sought to outline in this paper). It is a discursive regime, not a universal truth. Historians of medicine should by all means be encouraged to pursue the abundant visual objects in their field, and treat such objects in terms appropriate to the context of their production. A multiplicity of approaches is also to be encouraged. But they should do so with awareness of, and open candour towards, the historicity of the discourses around the visual from which their approaches derive. That is, they should be attentive to how their mindedness to the visual has been informed.[14]

But the response to such a warning in a moment now given to the empirical, the material, the "real" in the study of the history and culture of medicine, is to disqualify the study of representations as "merely" the interest of a subjective and therefore not transcendental history. W.J.T. Mitchell supported the view espoused by Cooter and Stein in the mid-1990s, observing that "representation (in memory, in verbal descriptions, in images) not only 'mediates' our knowledge (of slavery and of many other things), but obstructs, fragments, and negates that knowledge."[15] For him representations are not merely "objects representing" but an index (in the sense of C. S. Peirce) of the means by which representations are produced and received. Today's new functionalism seems to have moved towards the "real" in ways that question the very premises of theories of representation.

The shifts in the claims of the history and culture of medicine have not been as radical as those in recent literary interpretation. The new social history of medicine seems to have become a means of speaking about the reality that is merely mirrored in representations, while the real questions to be asked by the history and culture of medicine are understood to lie within clinical reality, biological empiricism, or even within the absolutes of social reality. Indeed, some of the directions that the medical humanities have taken departed from innovations in the biological sciences, such as the recent findings concerning the discovery of mirror neurons in neuroanatomy and the use of evolutionary theory as a model for the function of storytelling. But often this kind of interplay between medical humanities and the biological sciences comes to be an unquestioned, ahistorical approach that reifies the hypotheses of cutting-edge science without questioning them. This use of science should not be merely an expression of "discipline envy," as Marjorie Garber calls it when "literary studies has yearned to be and model itself on linguistics, anthropology, social science, natural science, psychoanalysis, sociology, history and various kinds of philosophy."[16] Rather, such approaches must value the methodologies of the humanities as part of an incorporation of the new sciences into the medical humanities rather than substituting a weak or reductive model of the sciences for the robust methods of the humanities.

As the medical humanities became a field within the new history of science that is more and more engaged with local, real, and material world aspects of health and illness, interest in representations has taken a backseat. In complicated ways we have returned to the negative attitudes of the first generation of medical historians in the late nineteenth century in regard to representations. I began to document such case studies decades ago in my book *Health and Illness: Images of Difference*.[17] Early medical historians in Imperial Germany had a great anxiety about the use of images, as they saw this initially as pandering to the public's desire for amusement. But what we have learned in our study of representations of health and illness over the past decades is that such images do not simply reflect an unmediated historical reality but rather reflect who we think we are in regard to the "real" past as much as how we imagine the past as an extension of ourselves. Indeed the dividing line between the history of medicine and the social study of medicine on the distinctions in the general field of the history of science and science studies seems to be on this fault line between interpretation and empiricism. The historian of science

Lorraine Daston commented on the distinctions in the general field of the history of science and science studies, or to put it into the language of the academy: the distinction between the soft and the hard disciplines.[18] She quotes the Harvard sociologist of technology

> Sheila Jasanoff, speaking qua president of the Society for the Social Studies of Science, [who] recently complained of a "somewhat one-sided love affair" with the history of science and a certain "jitteriness about being caught out in risqué company [that] marks the hiring practices of our major history of science departments.[19]

Social scientists interested in science want the hard empiricism of history, while, according to Daston, "the discipline of history . . . in turn was in hot pursuit of cultural anthropology."

Is "soft" the new "hard" for history? Hardly. For the history of science—and Daston's own work is a good example of this—has moved toward the technology by which representations are generated or captured as central to this new, hard history of science. It is the study of images that provides the core for a rethinking of the history of science. In Lorraine Daston and Peter Galison's *Objectivity* the historical epistemology of the image and its means of generation are at the core. Using the history of the scientific image from anatomy to crystallography, from the Enlightenment to the twentieth century, they sketch a world in which the creation of images is the reflection of the creation of a self-understanding of science within the consciousness of the scientist and, in turn, shapes that consciousness. The scientist's goal is as much in the "techniques of shaping the self, as well as of picturing nature."[20] Yet the claims of this critique of representations still assume some type of objective correlative, whether in the real world or in the psyche of the scientist. The critique of the assumption of objective correlatives in the psyche of the scientist is clear; the absence of a theory of mind (even a socially based theory of mind) places the "picturing of nature" as a reflex of the psyche of the scientist as a free-floating signifier. "Picturing" is moved from being an individual act in an historical context to that of the collective self-labeled as scientists without much consideration of the mechanisms present. But present and universal they are. It is, as Peter Novick argued decades ago, the creation of an academic notion of objectivity out of the subjectivity of the historical agent.[21] But the creation of such subjectivity follows the rules of ego formation and is not the mere whim of individuals in their historical context. Thus the scientific atlas is both the origin of and the creation of a scientific objectivity that defines the scope of evidence for the historian of science. But as historians we have to ask what psychological need such a creation fulfills.

While this new history of science with its bent toward a material (read: technological) world orientation is as much of a construct, of course, as the biologization of literary study through the application of evolutionary psychology or genetics, it is what is perceived as fashionable in 2010. Daston ends her account with the same problem that Cooter and Stein recognized in the field of medical representations, that the approaches of the history and the social study of science "are contingent to a certain time and place yet valid for certain purposes."[22] The history of medicine has moved in this direction; new models have appeared; old objects have been abandoned as they seem polluted by outmoded models of evidence and interpretation. The young Turks of the last generation have become the dons of this age; they must be swept away and their questions abandoned. Daston imagines a solution:

> . . . a new vision of what science is and how it works has yet to be synthesized from the rich but scattered and fragmented materials gathered by some twenty years of historicized history of science. The very practices that made that history possible militate against such a synthesis coming from the history of science itself. Science studies seems a still less likely candidate for the task. A new form of interdisciplinarity must be forged. Philosophy, anyone?[23]

Having just gone through the age of postmodern philosophical theory and a concomitant abandonment of the claims concerning falsifiability in the Popperian philosophy of science, philosophy seems a remote possibility for the future of the history and culture of medicine. Indeed the very claim of a line of demarcation between science and non-science, between medicine and quackery, comes to be called into question when the idea of a historically constituted epistemology is used.[24]

In the same issue Mario Biagioli noted that "the disciplinary predicament of science studies offers a useful vantage point for reconsidering some of the recent debates on the crisis of the humanities and the university."[25] For him the rupture between science and the humanities is post-Kuhnian with the now easy (his claim) political critique of science. At the conclusion of his essay, he presents a menu of options for what could be done to improve the interface between science and the humanities in the near future. He too demands a rethinking of the function of the study of visual images in science, including a departure from the study of medical images. His sixth bullet point reads:

> Science, visuality, imaging techniques, and so on. Such analyses should not be limited to the relationship between canonical art and canonical science (for example, Leonardo and anatomy) but expanded to encompass the study of the widespread production and role of all sorts of imaging techniques in science (both still and moving images). They could also venture in the direction of science-based art, like bio-art and tissue art.[26]

Is this the new aestheticism? Hard science now turned into the object of art galleries? In a real sense this simply echoes the new materialism: it replicates without questioning the image and its relationship to the very claims of science. Not surprisingly, any critique of the division between the soft and the hard approaches to the interface between the humanities and the real history of medicine looks at the image as the source for the study of the local, of the empirical, of technology and art; the cultural history of medical images, in this account, merely studies representations with their global meaning without much attention to the context or the history of the specific. This is Cooter and Stein's general point but is also echoed in Biagioli's as well as Daston's (and Galison's) critique. Yet this debate, which is inherent to the question of a new history of medicine, seems to be a recapitulation of what the study of images in the history and culture of medicine has been since the 1970s. Foucauldian globalism vs. the detailed study of the specific; the analysis of the epistemic vs. the concern with the detail; historical sociology or social study of science (whether Foucault or Latour) vs. "real" history. All center on readings of representations as key to rather than illustrative of Mitchell's problems of visual hermeneutics. Yet the very questions of the categories that Biagioli envisions as expanding the study of images point out the boundary question every more clearly. Where does the history of medical images end and the employment of such images in the world of art or at least in the world of the art gallery begin? Must we not ask questions about the constitution of a rapprochement between art and science but rather question the very selling of both? What does this employment of science in art and art as science tell us about discipline envy in the arts and the sciences? Can we see a clear line between the furthering of such art by foundations such as the Wellcome Trust in London and the sudden interest in the visual aspect of science as imported into the arts?

Why Is Learning to See Central to the Medical Humanities?

There is a need for a radical rethinking of the function of the study of representations in the medical humanities. The priority of representation in recent discussions within the field is evidence of this demand for its renewed attention. What position is open to us as critics of entire systems of visual and cultural representation in terms of a new or renewed epistemic? Where can we stand in terms of analyzing the reflection or distortion of the meanings associated with health and illness in the present world? The role of the study of medical (in the broadest sense) representations, or perhaps better, images of health and illness and their attendant social and cultural settings, needs to be addressed while acknowledging the new materialism and its claims about transcending its own cultural embeddedness. The function of representations (and those trained to study and analyze them) in the history of medicine is to knit the function of public and private representations with the continuities and discontinuities in attitudes and beliefs both within and beyond the health sciences. It is the frame for all empirical studies, as all such studies—whether epidemiological, genetic, developmental, social, or cultural—rely to one degree or the other on the analysis of representations. To study medical technology without understanding how its generation of representations is the key to its understanding is limited, as those working on fMRIs and genetics have shown; to study the representations without understanding the technology and the knowledge it generates is equally one-sided. To then examine the appropriateness of such images in the visual arts as a simple reflex of the interest in medicine in the world is naïve beyond belief. Today, medical images in art may be seen as a simple reaction to the increased importance of the health sciences in society, but they are also evidence for the appropriateness of art that explores the claims of the health sciences as to how they see and represent the world. Yet we must also understand the inherent limitations of our own positionality. Charles Taylor argues that:

> The tremendous prestige obtained by this kind of natural science in our culture produces a whole lot of phenomena, including a desire to confine medicine and practitioners to the things we really can be sure of. They fall into that category and leave the others outside. Or, it can take an imperialist form, where the belief is that the things that are dealt with, and let's say the self-interpreting fashion are actually largely illusory elements, that those dealing with illusions can find a way of dealing in terms of body chemistry.[27]

We engage with the world of medical representations not to show their duplicity or truth but to reveal their function in their historical context; we too are subject to this rule. We need to find a way to examine such representations by engaging with the debates about the meanings attached to representations and narratives in any given context as a way of bridging these growing gaps in the history and culture of medicine. By studying the claims about representations, we will come much closer to their underlying epistemic value in any given system. And, of equal importance, we can begin to understand the individual variants in or to these values. The study of representations thus is a paramount means of examining both collective and personal responses to cultural notions of health and illness, disease and healing, as well as to the institutions from the hospital to the advertising agencies engaged in these worlds.

The Case Studies

The case studies in this volume present a series of problems of seeing health and disease in the health sciences in the early twenty-first century. They examine in detail certain problems that reveal underlying continuities or ruptures in meaning within the health sciences. All of them rely on images, sometimes visual images, sometimes literary images, often medical images that frame the specific problem in ways that are not transparent. The historian of philosophy Robert Pippin observes that:

> Most everyone is willing to concede that the concepts by which we explain and evaluate our experience are "historically conditioned" in some sense. That ancient authors do not seem to recognize what Christian metaphysicians call the will, or that British philosophy of the 18th century ties normative distinctions so much to the influence of the passions, or that Kantian moral psychology describes agency as paradigmatically the capacity to obey the dictates of pure practical reason, do not look either like mere changes in fashion or eternally accessible problems, "discovered" by chance at one time rather than another. It looks like such changes will all have to be explained in a way that is profoundly "historical." But, as noted, it is not controversial to concede something like this. As with everything else, the devil is in the details.[28]

The case studies in this volume are intended to provide alternative approaches to questions of health and illness by examining the devil in the details. They rely on the close examination of representations, primarily in texts available in the public sphere. These texts range from the scientific to the fictional. While each in its time has its own claim on veracity, what these case studies do is to cull the shifts and continuities in meanings that are present within each of the examples on offer, exploring each case in regard to a historical and cultural context using evidence generated by the humanities rather than its absolute truth or fiction. Pippin notes that

> an important question here is what difference it makes that these examples are fictional, from a work of art; what would change if they were real-life examples? . . . [O]ne essential reason for having to rely on fiction is the possibility opened up of knowing quite a bit more about the state of and changes in the inner experience of characters than would ever be possible in "real life."[29]

But the "ring of truth" that Pippin seeks in his examination of the details is present in different ways within the materials examined in these case studies. The end point of such examinations is to show how what seems to be a stable set of meanings at any historical moment is part of a set of negotiations about that ring of truth.

Beginning with a case study on what I have chosen to call the "health exception" in the debates about male circumcision from the ancient world to the present, I show how competing fields of meaning, from religion to medicine, provide alternative and often contradictory images of what health is and how it can become part of what in the end are cultural debates about the body. How such arguments change over time based on the function that the images they rely on shift can be seen in the meanings attributed to infant male circumcision.

How we are seen in the world is the topic of the second case study on the meanings of authenticity in the arena of face transplantation. Here an evolving technical ability to alter the body comes with the baggage of what that body is supposed to look like. Popular accounts of face transplants as well as discussions with the surgeons who undertook them reveal a set of presuppositions about the authenticity of the body. What is "normal" is part of this discussion and the construction of the idea of the normal is central to any understanding of the health sciences.

The history of how we imagine what is human about human beings is to no little degree the history of posture, of our assumptions about upright and therefore healthy bodies. The case study of posture that follows traces the often contradictory idea of normal or healthy or beautiful posture in relationship to the history of disability and illness and disfigurement. Such contradictions and ambiguities can be found in the transnational history of the obese body.

Obesity is a central category for the discussion of illness or at least the etiology of illness in our time. Looking at its history in China, we can see how Western attitudes toward the image of the Chinese come to be part of the medical history of this category in the nineteenth and twentieth centuries. Obese bodies are real in the world, but the meanings attached to them have historical as well as cultural significance.

Pain, too, has such a history, and most importantly it has a history of being "seen," whether as a physiological or as a psychological experience. The image of pain—or perhaps better stated, of the way that pain is imagined—is part of its complex history in medicine and in art. But it is not just the body that is shaped by our images; the mind too shapes and is shaped by them.

If we examine the literature on the meanings associated with madness, here as a cultural statement of attitudes toward the widest scope of mental illness, we can understand that debates that appear to be about the status of mental illness are often about its meanings. This is most evident in the next case study, of a new category of mental illness coined officially in 2013, "self-harm," and how medicine projects the existence of such categories into the historical past in order to show that they are not bound in time and space and, therefore, are "real." Such illnesses are real, as this volume shows, even when their meanings are constantly shifting.

Certainly the history of the image of scientific racism, so very discredited because of the excesses of the Holocaust, has a history. But even in Germany, where that history is most acute, the debates about race have resurfaced, as they also resurfaced in the health sciences in the twenty-first century. How they are used and what they are taken to mean is the focus of this case.

The final essay is on the image of death. Here the idea of death in Western literature can be shown to be shaped by a series of confrontations in Western theology around its very meaning. Is death a closing of life, or is it an opening to a new life? This question colors much of our understanding of the end of life in contemporary Western culture, as the medical meaning of death is highly determined by its cultural representation.

To help focus the debates reflected in each of the case studies I have appended a set of questions. These are intended to help further reflection on the images analyzed and materials presented.

All of these case studies have the aim of illustrating how complex the questions raised in the medical humanities can be as they reflect on disciplinary approaches to such problems as well as the function that such cases can have within professional education. They are intended to be exemplary and will, I believe, show not so much how we can recuperate the humanities through such new applications but rather how the generation of knowledge is dependent on multiple and often contradictory approaches to the basic questions asked internally within the humanities and in fields such as the medical humanities. This book will not resolve the debates about the narrow question of the value of the humanities, but it will show you as a student of the medical humanities how the fault line often felt between the humanities and the health sciences is really a permeable boundary that enhances both—indeed may illustrate that there is no real boundary at all.

Notes

1. Evidence-based medicine is a concept coined by Gordon Guyatt at McMaster University in 1992 that sought to use the scientific evidence base to inform particular clinical decisions. See Milos Jenicek, "Epidemiology, Evidence-Based Medicine, and Evidence-Based Public Health," *Journal of Epidemiology* 7 (1997): 187–197 and Jane Macnaughton, "Medical Humanities' Challenge to Medicine," *Journal of Evaluation in Clinical Practice* 17 (2011): 927–932.
2. Charles Taylor, "Toward a Hermeneutical Conception of Medicine: A Conversation with Charles Taylor by Franco A. Carnevale and Daniel Weinstock," *Journal of Medicine and Philosophy* 36 (2011): 436–445, here 444.
3. Cited by Stanley Joel Reiser, "The Science of Diagnosis: Diagnostic Technology" in W. F. Bynum and Roy Porter, eds., *Companion Encyclopedia of the History of Medicine*, 2 vols., (London: Routledge,1993), 826–851, here Vol. 2, 829.
4. Hans-Georg Gadamer, *Truth and Method*, Trans. Garrett Barden and John Cumming. (New York: Seabury Press, 1975), 282.
5. Andrew Delbanco, *College: What it Was, Is, and Should Be* (Princeton: Princeton University Press, 2012), 96.
6. Ibid., 99.
7. Charles Taylor, "Self-interpreting Animals," *Philosophical Papers*: Vol. 1: *Human Agency and Language* (Cambridge, England: Cambridge University Press, 1985): 45–76; "Interpretation and the Sciences of Man," In *Interpretive Social Science: A Second Look* (Berkeley: University of California Press, 1987): 33–81.
8. See in particular the essays by Havi Hannah Carel, "Phenomenology as a Resource for Patients," *Journal of Medicine and Philosophy* 37(2012): 96–113 and "Phenomenology and its Application in Medicine," *Theoretical Medicine and Bioethics* 32 (2011): 33–46.
9. Jürgen Habermas, *The Future of Human Nature*, trans., Hella Beister, Max Pensky and William Rehg (Cambridge: Polity Press, 2003).

10. Marshall Hall, *The Principles of Diagnosis*. 2nd edition. (New York: Appelton, 1834), 31.
11. P. E. Baldry, *The Battle Against Heart Disease* (Cambridge: Cambridge University Press, 1971), 55.
12. Reiser, *Science of Diagnosis*, 828.
13. Roger Cooter and Claudia Stein, "Coming into Focus: Posters, Power, and Visual Culture in the History of Medicine," *Medizinhistorisches Journal* 42 (2007): 180–209. See also Jane Macnaughton, "Seeing Ourselves: Interpreting the Visual Signs of Illness," in Martyn Evans, et al., eds., *Medical Humanities Companion*. Volume One: *Symptom* (Oxford: Radcliffe Publishing, 2009), 71–85.
14. Ibid., 205.
15. W.J.T. Mitchell, *Picture Theory* (Chicago: University of Chicago Press, 1994), 188.
16. Marjorie Garber, *Academic Instincts* (Princeton: Princeton University Press, 2000), 66.
17. Sander L. Gilman, *Health and Illness: Images of Difference* (London: Reaktion Books, 1995).
18. Lorraine Daston "Science Studies and the History of Science," *Critical Inquiry* 35 (2009): 798–813.
19. Ibid., 798.
20. Lorraine Daston and Peter Galison, *Objectivity* (Cambridge: Zone Books, 2007), 363.
21. Peter Novick, *That Noble Dream: The Objectivity Question and the American Historical Profession* (Cambridge: Cambridge University Press, 1988).
22. Daston, 813.
23. Ibid., 813. This is a continuation of her argument in her earlier essay "'Baconian Facts', Academic Civility and the Prehistory of Objectivity," *Annals of Scholarship* 8 (1991): 337-364.
24. See Dirk Rupnow, Veronika Lipphardt, Jens Thiel and Christina Wessely, eds., *Pseudowissenschaft: Konzeptionen von Nichtwissenschaftlichkeit in der Wissenschaftsgeschichte* (Frankfurt am Main: Suhrkamp, 2008).
25. Mario Biagioli, "Postdisciplinary Liaisons: Science Studies and the Humanities," *Critical Inquiry* 35(2009): 816–32, 816.
26. Ibid., 832.
27. Taylor, *Hermeneutical Conception*, 437.
28. Robert Pippin, "'Philosophy is its own time comprehended in thought,'" *Topoi* (2006) 25:85–90, here 87.
29. Ibid., 90.

Questions

Why does there seem to be a battle between science and the humanities in higher education?

Are there really "two cultures in the intellectual life of the whole of western society," the sciences and the humanities, as the British novelist and scientist C. P. Snow claimed in his 1959 Rede Lecture? (http://s-f-walker.org.uk/pubsebooks/2cultures/Rede-lecture-2-cultures.pdf)

What is a representation, and how does it relate to lived experience?

How do representations function in the role of the humanities in the study of medicine, health, and illness?

London / Atlanta Summer 2013

Case One

Circumcision: Religion and Health

Problems: What happens when religion and health compete or are allied? The United States is the nation in which infant male circumcision is most widely accepted and practiced, but for health rather than for religious reasons. Immediately after birth infant male children have their foreskins surgically removed. The United States has the greatest rate even though the number of male infants circumcised for any reason has declined today to about 55 percent from a high of almost 80 percent during the 1970s and '80s In Europe, in contrast, only 10 percent of boys are circumcised. In what contexts does circumcision occur as a health practice, and what are the implications of health-related/medically indicated circumcision for the health sciences?

Religion and Health?

The Princeton cultural anthropologist James A. Boon has argued "foreskins are facts—cultural facts whether removed or retained. Absent versus present, prepuces have divided many religions, politics, and ritual persuasions. . . . (Non)circumcision involves signs separating an 'us' from a 'them' entangled in various discourses of identity and distancing."[1] It is this theme—that circumcision is a cultural fact that provides meaning when there is a confrontation between traditions and peoples that advocate or disparage the practice—that I wish to pursue in this chapter. I will trace multiple religious and medical approaches to circumcision to illustrate that each continually occupy and create cultural meanings for and from this procedure.

Circumcision, as Boon has shown, can be seen as a case study, as an index of difference in societies, but it can also take on nuances that those societies give it in regard to other, highly valued arenas of the production of other forms of meaning. Foreskins are thus not only cultural facts, they are the space for the accretion of multiple cultural connotations depending on the salience of other systems of value in a given society at a given moment.[2] Certainly one of the major points of confusion in the history of circumcision is the elision (and now the assumption) that the meaning of this practice within religion is coterminous with that in medicine. These are two different worlds of meaning. Although they constantly borrow one from the other, this process of borrowing is always accompanied by a shift in the meaning ascribed to that which is borrowed. Similarly, "medical testimony" before a court is only superficially related to medicine, as it draws on the status of medicine in support of its forensic claims, but is ruled by radically different meanings. This is also true in the function of circumcision within the worlds of theology and medicine, even though this distinction is not always clearly the case.

The Debate about Circumcision in the Twenty-First Century

The recent debates on circumcision in the West (specifically Europe and the United States) have made this conflation of the medical meaning of circumcision and all other possible meanings of the practice evident in an interesting and often conflicted way.[3] Is circumcision a religious practice that incidental has health benefits, or is it a medical practice sometimes undertaken for religious purposes? In August 2012, the American Academy of Pediatrics reversed its stand on infant male circumcision. Originally in 1971 they had stated, "There are no valid medical indications for circumcision in the neonatal period."[4] By 1999 they began to waffle: "Existing scientific evidence demonstrates potential medical benefits of newborn male circumcision; however, these data are not sufficient to recommend routine neonatal circumcision."[5] In August, 2012 there was no longer any hesitation:

> Systematic evaluation of English-language peer-reviewed literature from 1995 through 2010 indicates that preventive health benefits of elective circumcision of male newborns outweigh the risks of the procedure. . . . Although health benefits are not great enough to recommend routine circumcision for all male newborns, the benefits of circumcision are sufficient to justify access to this procedure for families choosing it and to warrant third-party payment for circumcision of male newborns.[6]

From no health benefit to sufficient health benefit, from religious practice to medical intervention, from discouraging to encouraging in less than fifty years.

In May of 2012, the equivalent German organizations (the Dachverband der Kinder- und Jugendmedizinischen Gesellschaften and the Berufsverband der Kinder- und Jugendärzte) had stated exactly the opposite. Their argument that circumcision violates the bodily integrity of the infant—as well as putting the infant's health at risk—was supported by a German court ruling later that year banning the procedure for these reasons. The case brought before the court involved the circumcision of a four-year-old Muslim boy that was performed by a doctor at the parents' request. Complications occurred with the operation that resulted in the Cologne public prosecutor charging the doctor with the grievous bodily harm of the infant. The district court, hearing the case in the first instance, acquitted the doctor on the grounds that there was parental consent and that he had performed the procedure as a ritual act based on Islam.[7] The first court's position supports a view of circumcision as a procedure to be encouraged as a prophylaxis; the later ruling sees it as a nonmedical procedure that is harmful and violates the infant's human rights.

What is fascinating about this debate is that it takes place within institutions of medicine, specifically pediatrics, in cultures that place the highest premium on medicine providing objective truths, especially in their application of medical knowledge within judicial processes. National medical organizations do debate the status of procedures, for example, raising and lowering cutoffs for hypertension, approving and then not approving medications or treatments, for example, mammography, mastectomy, Prostate Specific Antigen testing, and these debates do take different turns in different national settings. Rarely are these debates the locus of the intersection of religious practice and evidence-based medicine.

That the West moves from a culture of religious belief (including concerns about circumcision) to one of a culture of science in the hundred years leading up to the European Enlightenment is a commonplace understanding, best articulated in terms of the warfare between "theology" and "science."[8] "Theology" is a specific religious claim or structure rather than a religious belief itself; while "science" more and more in the course of the nineteenth century comes to focus on medicine as its litmus test for acceptable authority. But, as we shall see, this movement toward medicine as a litmus test actually occurs long before the nineteenth century, when a system with a cultural acceptance of circumcision within religious practice comes into conflict with a system that denigrates it but has a powerful autonomous medical tradition. This seems very different from the pattern that Boon found on Java where two religious systems, one circumcising, one not, were (and remain) in conflict. They define the line of demarcation between "civilized" and "primitive," between believer and non-believer. As we shall see in asymmetrical systems, such as those where science trumps theology, the acceptance or rejection of the practice is often colored by the status of circumcision in medicine rather than theology.

A Complex History

Boon's characterization of the conflicted meaning of circumcision traces a long and fraught history. Historically, discussions of circumcision have included female as well as male genital cutting.[9] In this case study, I focus on male genital cutting, although I shall mention the generally negative consensus about female genital cutting that colors present debates in the West. While a multitude of societies have practiced and continue to practice male circumcision (the procedure is documented as early as the twenty-third century BC in Egypt), its place in contemporary debates is focused on its continued ritual practice in Judaism and Islam. Uha, in the twenty-third century BC, describes a mass Egyptian ritual circumcision of future priests and boasts of his ability to stoically endure the pain: "When I was circumcised, together with one hundred and twenty men . . . there was none thereof who hit out, there was none thereof who was hit, and there was none thereof who scratched and there was none thereof who was scratched."[10] This was a religious test linked to the coming of age of young men destined for the priesthood. No discussion of any medical efficacy is present, even given the wide range of Egyptian medical papyri. Circumcision is defined as a religious act even though, or perhaps because, it involves amputating a part of the body and it is an action often depicted as part of Egyptian medicine.

To those who practice it, infant male circumcision is a powerful sign of group identity: it defines the community of the ancient Egyptians and later of the Jews and Muslims who adopt it. (Jews must perform the ritual on the eighth day after birth, while Muslims can and do circumcise up to the fourteenth year of life. In general the overall focus on this procedure in the context of the health exception has been on the circumcision of infants. There are exceptions such as adult circumcision and also circumcision for adults converting to Judaism; and even if the person had been circumcised at birth (as a gentile) some blood has to be drawn to validate the conversion.) This communitarian view has a powerful resonance in Jewish history after the destruction of the second Temple, when it becomes the primary sign of Jewish identity. Even slaves must be circumcised, indicating the significance of male circumcision as one of the central communitarian acts defining the bounds of the group. As in Genesis 17:13-14:

> He that is born in thy house, and he that is bought with thy money, must needs be circumcised; and My covenant shall be in your flesh for an everlasting covenant. . . . And the uncircumcised male who is not circumcised in the flesh of his foreskin, that soul shall be cut off from his people; he hath broken My covenant.

Temple Judaism practices the ritual of infant male circumcision as a religious imperative, needing only a divine rationale for its undertaking.

As the world of the Jews became more and more Hellenized in the second-century BC, the claim of a communitarian identity through infant male circumcision is contested. Indeed, this is the very moment where its absolute necessity as the defining action for membership in the religious community is made paramount. Thus in the land of Israel circumcision is a problem for some Jews, as we read in 1 Maccabees 1:15-1:15. where such Jews during the first century BC "removed the marks of circumcision, and abandoned the holy covenant. They joined with the Gentiles and sold themselves to do evil."

Medicine and Circumcision

That circumcision is condemned in Greco-Roman antiquity is clear. In the Satyricon, Petronius has Cito says, "Circumcise us, that we may appear to be Jews."[11] Tacitus in the *Histories* observes that the Jews "have instituted circumcising the genitals in order to be distinguished by this difference." It is a custom that Tacitus finds "base and abominable, persisting due to their depravity."[12] But it is also clear that circumcised males sought out the most advanced medical techniques of the day to remove this sign of circumcision. Surgery, as we read in the work of Aulus Cornelius Celsus (25 BC–AD 50) is undertaken to restore the foreskin and therefore reconstitute a healthy body:

> But in one who has been circumcised the prepuce is to be raised from the underlying penis mound the circumference of the glans by

> means of a scalpel. This is not so very painful, for once the margin has been freed, it can be stripped up by hand as far back as the pubes, nor in doing so is there any bleeding, The prepuce thus freed is again stretched forwards beyond the glans: next cold water effusions are freely used, and a plaster is applied round to repress severe inflammation. And for the following days the patient is to fast until nearly overcome by hunger lest satiety excite that part. When the inflammation has ceased, the penis should be bandaged from the pubes to the corona; over the glans the plaster is applied with the other end of the probe. This is done in order that the lower part [between the corona and pubic area] may agglutinate, whilst the upper part [the new foreskin covering the glans] heals without adhering.[13]

Celsus records these surgical procedures for elongating or replicating the male foreskin, for he sees this as one of the roles that medicine plays in reconfiguring the male body as a healthy one, able to enter into the social activities in the Gymnasium.[14] Thus out of parochial Jews, cosmopolitan Greco-Romans were made.

Indeed in time circumcision came to be banned among the Jews by Antiochus IV (215–164 BC). For as Josephus writes:

> Menelaus and the sons of Tobias were distressed, and retired to Antiochus, and informed him that they were desirous to leave the laws of their country, and the Jewish way of living according to them, and to follow the king's laws, and the Grecian way of living. Wherefore they desired his permission to build them a Gymnasium at Jerusalem. And when he had given them leave, they also hid the circumcision of their genitals, that even when they were naked they might appear to be Greeks. Accordingly, they left off all the customs that belonged to their own country, and imitated the practices of the other nations.[15]

In other words, the religious practice of the Jews came in conflict with the attitudes of the Greeks and Romans toward any "disfiguring" of the body with as potent a result as Boon saw on Java. The dominant political and cultural elite saw the act as barbaric mutilation without any redeeming features whatsoever. How could one justify the act except from a reactive, conservative theological position such as the one taken by the Maccabees?

The Jewish philosopher Philo of Alexandria (20 BC–AD 50) wrote in this strongly Hellenistic culture where, according to Josephus (in his *Against Apion*), the Alexandrian Apion derided the practice of circumcision. Philo in *De specialibus legibus* advocated for the practice, noting that it was a prophylaxis against diseases of the penis—"preventive of a painful disease, and of an affliction difficult to be cured, which they call a carbuncle,"—and also promoted the well-being of the individual and assured fertility.[16] Circumcision may be a Jewish ritual that alters the body, but it also presents a health advantage. The Greek historian Herodotus (484–425 BC) (2:37) dismisses this claim when he writes about the Egyptians (and those who learned circumcision from them) that they "practice circumcision for the sake of purity, considering it better to be pure than comely."[17] Here we see the power of what I am calling the "health exception," the evocation of medicine, for good or for ill, in regard to a practice that had been considered purely religious. The health exception works in both directions: it is seen as recuperative, preventing, or curing, or it is seen as destructive and harmful because it disrupts the natural beauty of the male body and disfigures it, a sign of illness. The health exception exists when there is no consensus about the practice of infant male circumcision in a society with competing values and with a strong medical tradition.

Circumcision and Identity

Modernity, at least in the Western Diaspora, came to regard infant male circumcision as the key marker of a Jewish religious identity. As Spinoza in his *Tractatus Theologico-Politicus* (1670) noted: "the sign of circumcision is, as I think so important that I could persuade myself that it alone would preserve the nation forever."[18] Yet for Christians of Spinoza's age, circumcision had been dismissed by Paul as inherently Jewish and, therefore, after the rise of Christianity, not defining the universal claims of Christianity but only the parochial views of the Jews. It was a Noahide law, pertaining only to the Jews. Boon comments that "at the mention of circumcision the Balinese dike of tolerance collapsed; the outpouring in Indonesian went something like this: What are they doing that here for? That's the trouble with Muslims, too fanatical."[19] Certainly the "dike of tolerance" in Europe was regularly breached when circumcision was raised in the context of Jewish practice.

The view that the Jews, again to quote Boon, were "too fanatical" about circumcision was espoused by the Church Fathers, Eusebius, and Origen and continued through the Renaissance (Erasmus was opposed to the practice) and through the Reformation (as was Luther). One has the body one is born with, said the Church Fathers at the Council of Jerusalem in AD 50, waiving Jewish practices such as circumcision. But they did not forbid it, and even today Coptic Christians (living in a Muslim culture that does require circumcision) practice this rite. Yet most Christians agreed (and agree) with Immanuel Kant in his *Religion Within the Boundaries of Mere Reason* (1793):

> The subsequent discarding of the corporeal sign which served wholly to separate these people from others is itself warrant for the judgment that the new faith [Christianity], not bound to the statutes of the old, nor, indeed, to any statute at all, was to contain a religion valid for the world and not for one single people.[20]

By abandoning such practices one becomes universal and thus truly and authentically human. This view of a Jewish particularism defined by circumcision is held even by liberals such as the Italian physician Paolo Mantegazza, clearly, if mockingly, an advocate of hygiene:

> Circumcision is a shame and an infamy; and I, who am not in the least anti-Semitic, who indeed have much esteem for the Israelites, I who demand of no living soul a profession of religious faith, insisting only upon the brotherhood of soap and water and of honesty, I shout and shall continue to shout at the Hebrews, until my last breath: Cease mutilating yourselves: cease imprinting upon your flesh an odious brand to distinguish you from other men; until you do this, you cannot pretend to be our equal. As it is, you, of your own accord, with the branding iron, from the first days of your lives, proceed to proclaim yourselves a race apart, one that cannot, and does not care to, mix with ours.[21]

While circumcision is seen as creating a communitarian identity, this is seen negatively, separating the Jews from their peers.

It is the health exception that is the means by which ritual practice is accepted or rejected in Western Enlightened society, and it impacts on the ritual practice and meaning of the procedure within religious communities. Within eighteenth-century European science, following the new scientific view of the inheritance of acquired characteristics, the assumption was that Jewish males could be born without a foreskin—that they were often aposthetic. This marked them as inherently different from other groups and was part of the arguments that were eventually used to focus in on racial differences between Jews and other races. According to Johann David Michaelis, the noted Orientalist of the German Enlightenment, it is true that the Jew, like the ape, can be born circumcised. But Michaelis interprets this anomaly in no way as a sign of the higher status of the Jew. Michaelis would consider circumcision as evidence of higher status only if such a condition gave a specific advantage to those born circumcised. And for Michaelis, living in the midst of a world that firmly believed in masturbation as the origin of a myriad number of physical and psychological ailments, he relies on the understanding that circumcision has no curative powers to reverse or prevent illnesses due to masturbation as an argument against its conferral of any advantage. Circumcision, he states, is not a cure for masturbation. Those born without a prepuce are no better off than anyone else. Michaelis argues that nature would have made the act of masturbation, a source of sin as well as a source of illness, completely impossible rather than dealing with it through aposthia. The Jew, Michaelis notes, following Philo, takes those born circumcised for especially holy men since they have a diminished sexual urge.[22] We, he implies, know better. One must note here that in the Hadith, the written accounts of Mohammed's life and observation, he too was born without a foreskin, as a sign of his perfection. For Islam, infant male circumcision comes to be seen as one of the practices known as *fitra*, acts considered to be those of a refined person. There is no detailed discussion of Islam in any of these Enlightenment discussions of the pitfalls of circumcision as it is a hammer used specifically to characterize European Jewry.

The liberal anthropologist Johann Friedrich Blumenbach argued for the existence of congenital circumcision in his study of the sexual drive (1781). It is important to note that Blumenbach was a strong opponent of the polygenetic theory of the races, which saw the races as inherently different. (Although, he also believed that Jews—or, at least, their skulls—were immediately and incontrovertibly identifiable as distinct.) He was also a strong advocate (as were most of his contemporaries) of the view that acquired characteristics could be inherited. If Jews (and others) circumcised their children, it was reasonable to expect that some "boys in the orient are born circumcised."[23] That this marker was understood as a marker of Jewish identity in all cases can be seen in Friedrich Schiller's ironic treatment of his "Jewish" character Moritz Spiegelberg in his first play, *The Robbers* (1782). Schiller intends to show Spiegelberg's duplicity by having Spiegelberg deny his Jewish identity. The character is made to refer to himself as having been "miraculously born circumcised."[24] His denial of the religious origin of his circumcision is a comment on the nature of the Jew, seen, at least by Schiller, as mendacious.[25]

Modern Biology and Circumcision

Charles Darwin left the question of circumcision and identity open in his 1868 study of *The Variation of Animals and Plants under Domestication.* In asking the question of whether mutilations or injuries can be acquired, he observes: "With respect to Jews, I have been assured by three medical men of the Jewish faith that circumcision, which has been practiced for so many ages, has produced no inherited effect; Blumenbach, on the other hand, asserts that in Germany Jews are often born in a condition rendering circumcision difficult, so that a name is there applied to them signifying 'born circumcised.'"[26] Yet later Darwinians have a very specific take on this: Hastings Tweedy, president of the Section of Obstetrics of the Royal Academy of Medicine in Ireland in 1920, observed that he "had never satisfied himself that the craze for circumcision was justifiable. According the laws of evolution the foreskin must have been greatly needed by the human race or it would not have persisted."[27] Circumcision is a "natural" (and therefore healthy) occurrence among the Jews . . . unless it is not.

This debate about the special relationship between Jews and ritual circumcision and the health exception is reflected in the Verein der Reformfreunde (Society for the Friends of Reform) in Frankfurt, which in 1843 said that ritual infant male circumcision was neither a religious obligation nor a symbolic act.[28] This was in response to the February 8, 1843, finding of the Frankfurt Public Health authority that circumcision had to be carried out under medical supervision. With the expanding role of medicine came further opposition; certain ritual aspects of Jewish circumcision such as *metzitzah* (drawing the blood from the circumcision wound through sucking) were deemed unhygienic (Katz 1998: 337–402). Outbreaks of syphilis and tuberculosis from 1805 to 1865 were blamed on the ritual circumcisers. Many reformers thus advocated modifying metzitzah using a sponge or a glass tube. But the end result of concerns over hygiene and deformation was that ritual circumcision was less and less undertaken by acculturated Jews in Central and Western Europe.

The idea that the circumcised were inherently different because they were marked as Jewish dominates the nineteenth-century discussion. Through the Enlightenment, discussions of such religious practices seemed to be colored by debates about their medical efficacy, but these is never neutral as specific attitudes toward the Jews seem always to define this debate. As an anonymous author stated in the leading

German pediatric journal, *Journal für Kinderkrankheiten*, in 1872: "The circumcision of Jewish children has been widely discussed in the medical press as is warranted with topics of such importance. But it is usually discussed without the necessary attention to details and the neutrality that it deserves. Indeed, it has not been free of fanatic anti-Semitism."[29] No discussion of circumcision within medicine is without an ideological perspective. This prefigures the discussion that James Boon has concerning Peter Charles Remondino's 1891 view of the "intolerant uncircumcision in a history of totalitarian prejudices too notorious to need reviewing."[30]

The reintroduction of the surgical reconstruction of the foreskin in the mid-nineteenth century is seen as a political act by Johann Friedrich Dieffenbach in his classic handbook *Die operative Chirurgie* (1845):

> One must understand me correctly. I present such methods only for their physiological-surgical principles and to illustrate Celsus' idea of the extension of the prepuce out of luxury, belief, shame, or politics. It would be a denigration of the art [of surgery] if in this manner bachelors are created like virgins through the reconstitution of the hymen, about which one writer so pointedly said: 'a fine operation!' Both are a morbid mockery of humanity from the practice of the oriental slave trader."[31]

Here the negative health exception takes precedence such operations are not medically necessary but rather serve to draw medicine itself into disrepute. Dieffenbach believed that doctors who perform this surgery are quite aware that they are indulging patients with an aesthetic procedure that has no medical value.

By the mid-nineteenth century the terms of the definition of the practice centered about the health exception. This discussion was part of a more general medical debate about whether the Jews, by their ritual practice or eugenic selection, were healthier or sicker than other groups. Thus in 1890, John S. Billings, the head of the Library of the Surgeon General's Office in Washington, persuaded the Census Bureau to undertake a census (the only one ever) of the racial diseases of a specific group—the Jews. He queries, "Are these differences due to race characteristics, properly so-called, to original and inherited differences in bodily organization, or are they, rather, to be attributed to the customs, habits, and modes of life of the two classes of people?"[32] Answering this, Billings noted that when Jews became integrated into American culture they showed their inherent racial degeneracy in spite of their ritual hygienic practices such as circumcision. In regard to circumcision, the argument is heard on both sides. In 1860 a London practitioner, Dr. Fowler, writing in the *Lancet* could claim the complete efficacy of circumcision in combating one of the most widespread etiologies of illness of the time, masturbation:

> Has the operation of circumcision any effect in diminishing the habit or practice of onanism amongst the male children and the young lads of the Jewish community? Practising in a neighbourhood where this community abounds, I do not remember ever having had either a confessed or even a suspected case of this description amongst our Hebrew brethren. I wish I could say the same respecting juvenile Christians.[33]

The claim is that circumcision by definition leads to the amelioration of the practice of masturbation and thus to its consequences.

One of the only persistent factors in debates on circumcision is the coexistence of extreme opinions on such efficacy. Additionally, circumcision is often debated alongside issues of public health. Advocacy for the procedure in both cases is based on a positive health exception. Indeed, the American physician Peter Charles Remondino, so well discussed by Boon, projects his nineteenth-century fascination with circumcision as hygiene into the world of the Egyptians: "In ancient Egypt . . . the nobility, royalty, and the higher warrior class seem to have adopted circumcision as well, either as a hygienic precaution or as an aristocratic prerogative and insignia" (Remondino 1891: iii). While arguments relying on the health exception to show that the dangers of circumcision persist, the image of the health exception that Remondino successfully argues for in late nineteenth-century America contributes to the creation of a climate that makes the United States into a circumcising culture. In the 1920s, a debate in the Royal Academy of Medicine in Ireland saw a Dr. Solomons defend the practice of circumcision: "most educated people ask to have their sons circumcised." It helps "in preventing masturbation." Circumcision is advised as "a real help to the weakest spot in the human character." The "ordinary schoolboy was not taught to keep himself clean." Solomons argued that the procedure did not require anesthesia: "in fact it was harmful." He also argued that syphilis is five times greater in the uncircumcised. Our Darwinian physician Hastings Tweedy argued the case against Solomons and stated that circumcision does not "reduce sexual desire." Dr. Tweedy also doubted Solomons's figures about prophylaxis against syphilis. He had seen fatal cases in circumcised patients, three caused by chloroform and one from hemorrhage (Report, 1920: 768). In the 1930s there was a debate in Great Britain on whether the government should require infant male circumcision, and arguments for medical intervention became central. One physician at the time held that "if the removal of the prepuce lessens the incidence of syphilis . . . then circumcision is surely a duty in all cases."[34] Such claims were regularly made throughout the nineteenth century, advocating circumcision as a preventative against a range of diseases from the evils of masturbation to sexually transmitted diseases. Infant male circumcision is valuable because it has a positive health impact unless, of course, it doesn't.

Circumcision and Illness Today

The debates about circumcision as a prophylaxis against syphilis (and other STIs) had been a staple of the late-nineteenth-century hygiene debates. Indeed, it lay at the center of why the United States became a medically circumcising culture (even with a decrease in rates today) while much of the rest of the Western world did not. These debates about circumcision were always countered with the claim that the very act of ritual circumcision actually transmitted syphilis and often caused death or impairment through the surgery itself. The clearest result after 150 years of debates about the efficacy of circumcision as a prophylaxis against infectious disease is the determination both anecdotally and epidemiologically that such a procedure has little or no effect on STI transmission in Western cultures. Indeed, the American practice of circumcision began during the late nineteenth century and continued with other medical rationales (for example, reduced cases of penile cancer and uterine cancer in sexual partners) after the introduction of antibiotics for the treatment of STIs. The practice of circumcision continues as a rationale for the reduction of cases of cervical cancer even after a specific vaccination protocol (Gardisil) is available for those forms of HPV that are antecedent to many of such cancers. Of course, the debate about what is in the best interest of the child resurfaces around this procedure, a three-course vaccination: does it place children at risk either from perceived or imaginary side effects from the vaccine? Does it place the child at risk for increased promiscuity because of the absence of risk from HPV infection?[35] The use of the vaccine is now generally accepted as a powerful force in reducing HPV infections in men and women, while the evidence for the efficacy of circumcision, considering the surgical risk, is more limited.

Health is primary in debates over circumcision, but what defines health differs from advocate to opponent. By the 1950s, another rethinking of the health exception is undertaken as the impact of Anna Freud's idea of the "best interest of the child" comes into contact with the promotion of the human rights that should be afforded the bodily integrity of the child. Infant (human) rights confronted another form of human right, that of communitarianism in the form of the rights of the religious community. (Here one must add that Anna's father, Sigmund, saw circumcision in terms of the health exception as a source of psychopathology in his account of the case of Little Hans in his *Analysis of a Phobia in a Five-year-old Boy* [1909].) Again and again, circumcision is attacked as the "rape of the phallus." The focus is on infant pain and bodily integrity, from the perspective of the best interest of the child.[36]

These negative medical evaluations of circumcision come to color its legal reception in Europe. A law on circumcision of boys was adopted in Sweden in 2001, in the aftermath of a 1997 Swedish Supreme Court decision holding "that ritual circumcision of a minor boy that was performed with parental consent was not punishable as assault" (Swedish Supreme Court 1997). This was the first law concerning circumcision passed in Europe following the end of the Third Reich.[37] The law is a set of medical directives and stipulates that only a licensed doctor may perform a circumcision on boys less than two months old and that a licensed doctor or certified anesthesiologist must be present; that the parents, if they share joint parental responsibility, must be in agreement about the procedure for the child; and "if possible, the boy himself should provide informed consent to be circumcised. The law states that regardless of age, a boy's wishes not to be circumcised should always be respected." (The court is careful not to define how is the boy's wish is to be ascertained and to see that this caveat does not set a precedent for minors' refusal of all sorts of medical procedures unless the procedure is not classified as medical.) While the question of agency seems to be paramount, the stated rationale was to reduce the risk of the procedure to the health of the infant.

The discussions in 2012 are no different. Opponents argue that male circumcision is bad because it violates the body, especially that of the infant, unless it has a medical rationale. Only when medically indicated is circumcision in the best interest of the child. Conversely, the argument goes: Infant male circumcision is good because it creates a powerful group identity, which is in the best interest of the child.

The latter argument is even more powerful when this group identity can also claim that circumcision confers positive health benefits. It is also the case that a negative impact on health can counter any communitarian claim. Thus the British NHS dropped newborn circumcision in 1949 in response to Douglas Gairdner, who opposed it in a widely quoted essay. Gairdner noted that the procedure was linked to sixteen deaths annually, although these were from the general anesthetics employed, not the circumcision itself.[38]

When in 1999 the issue of the parents' right to circumcise comes before British courts, it is the Muslim practice that is seen at putting the child at risk:

> Re "J" (child's religious upbringing and circumcision) said that circumcision in Britain required the consent of all those with parental responsibility, or the permission of the court, acting for the best interests of the child, and issued an order prohibiting the circumcision of a male child of a non-practicing Muslim father and non-practicing Christian mother with custody. The reasoning included evidence that circumcision carried some medical risk; that the operation would be likely to weaken the relationship of the child with his mother, who strongly objected to circumcision without medical necessity; that the child may be subject to ridicule by his peers as the odd one out and that the operation might irreversibly reduce sexual pleasure, by permanently removing some sensory nerves, even though cosmetic foreskin restoration might be possible. The court did not rule out circumcision against the consent of one parent.[39]

In Britain as well as on the Continent, the presence of a large and new Muslim community means that Muslims have become the litmus test for bad communitarian practices rather than Jews. The liberal consensus against "Islamic rituals" such as female genital cutting also easily extends itself to rituals such as infant male circumcision as a violation of human rights, as in the anti-Islam campaigner Hirsi Ali's 2004 short-lived opposition to the practice of infant male circumcision.[40]

An American Praxis

Yet in the United States, it remains a Jewish practice, and it continues to attract the attention of the health authorities. Recently in New York City, ritual metzitzah among ultra-orthodox Jews has been blamed for infant deaths from herpes. The New York City Board of Health passed a regulation on September 12, 2012, to require parental notification of risk, a demand that has been vociferously opposed by religious authorities who note that the procedure is never the cause of any possible danger to the health of the infant. According to the Board of Health about 3,600 male infants are circumcised with direct oral suction each year, and their risk of contracting herpes is estimated at roughly 1 in 4,000. The Centers for Disease Control and Prevention call the procedure unsafe and recommend against it. Indeed, some members of the Board of Health said they believed that requiring consent did not go far enough. "It's crazy that we allow this to go on," said Dr. Joel A. Forman, a professor of pediatrics at Mount Sinai School of Medicine. Again, the debates center on ritual as communitarian practice versus the health of the infant: "This process [demanded by the Board of Health] is being created without a shred of evidence," said Rabbi William Handler, one of a few ultra-Orthodox Jews who gathered outside the meeting in protest. "The city is lying, and slandering compassionate rabbis."[41] "They feel that if their child doesn't have the metzitzah, he is not Jewish, so this, to them, is the most important act that they can do for their son in life," said Dr. Kenneth I. Glassberg, the director of the division of pediatric urology at Morgan Stanley Children's Hospital at New York-Presbyterian. "Medically, I don't approve of it," he added of the oral contact, "but if you're asking me, 'Does it cause harm?' I haven't seen enough proof that it causes harm" (Otterman 2012). This is the problem with the health exception: since it argues theology against science, neither side can muster sufficient evidence to persuade the other.

It is the rather new concept of "health risk," rather than the transmission of infectious diseases, that is now invoked for and against the practice in New York. As Susan Bewley, professor of obstetrics, and Sarah Strandjord, professor of pediatrics, Kings College (London) argue:

> if neonatal circumcision is beneficial, it should be recommended for all (accepting that parents do not have to take the advice). If it is not beneficial (or risky or harmful), then society can either allow some leeway for parents to harm their infants (with or without medical collusion), or disallow it until boys are of an age to make their own decisions.[42]

This is a rather bold restatement of the role that the health exception plays in these arguments. In other words, health trumps group identity unless the group identity can draw on a health rationale. Sadly, this debate has never been separate from attitudes toward religious ritual. In the 1990s, the focus in Europe turned to Muslim ritual practice, especially in the British and German courts. Indeed the shades of Mantegazza's antireligious liberalism found as echoes in the opposition to practices such as female genital cutting have been easily extended to rituals such as infant male circumcision as violations of human rights, as Hirsi Ali claimed in 2004. Only when the health exception is advocated can there be an argument for an elective surgical procedure for infants and that has never been done for female genital cutting even within Islam.[43]

Thus the American Academy of Pediatrics's advocacy rests on an evaluation of a wide range of studies, but at its core are the CDC studies that argue for a radically reduced rate of HIV transmission in circumcised males in sub-Saharan Africa. But as one recent study claims:

> sub Saharan studies of circumcision benefit used in support of "universal" circumcision in Africa including infant circumcision have been subjected to critical re-analyses which indicate the benefit has been overstated: reporting relative risk reduction rather than the absolute risk reduction of only 1.3 percent in female to male HIV transmission while ignoring the 61 percent increase in male to female HIV transmission posed by circumcised males.[44]

And indeed the CDC Federal Register Notice proposal for universal circumcision in the United States, as advocated by Bewley and Strandjord, was recently withdrawn from the Web without explanation. This is not to say that circumcision may not reduce the risk of certain rates of disease, but as a rationale for its wider application, its efficacy in preventing the actual transmission of disease remains unproven even with recent claims in 2014 by the US president's emergency plan for Aids relief (Pepfar) and UNAids, which do not take into consideration the wide range of other parallel interventions that maybe reducing HIV transmissions in countries such as Uganda. The counter argument focusing on the human rights of the infant is also flawed, for medical and forensic arguments for vaccination, surgical, and therapeutic intervention—as well as forced blood transfusions that run counter to the interests of parents on religious grounds have been well documented over the past century. European pediatricians argue that the changes are purely culturally biased:

> Seen from the outside, cultural bias reflecting the normality of nontherapeutic male circumcision in the United States seems obvious, and the report's conclusions are different from those reached by physicians in other parts of the Western world, including Europe, Canada,

> and Australia. In this commentary, a different view is presented by non–US-based physicians and representatives of general medical associations and societies for pediatrics, pediatric surgery, and pediatric urology in Northern Europe. To these authors, only 1 of the arguments put forward by the American Academy of Pediatrics has some theoretical relevance in relation to infant male circumcision; namely, the possible protection against urinary tract infections in infant boys, which can easily be treated with antibiotics without tissue loss.[45]

Once you make the health exception, any communitarian argument against medical intervention is just as flawed.[46]

Certainly the debates about this question, so substantially raised in the proposal to make it "unlawful to circumcise, excise, cut, or mutilate the whole or any part of the foreskin, testicles, or penis" of anyone seventeen or younger in San Francisco in the spring of 2011, aired a litany of "human rights" claims, from freedom of religion to the question of bodily integration to the problem of informed consent when such practices are performed on infants. Underlying this attempt at legally barring circumcision is the stated assumption that such interventions harm the infant's body by severing nerves in the penis. The influential Los Angeles Rabbi David Wolpe read this as an anti-Semitic attack on religious freedom: "Some involved are simply opposed to religion (there are after all some misguided Jews arguing for the ban as well), some wish to target both Muslims and Jews. But can anyone doubt that there are anti-circumcision advocates who seize on this as a chance to hurt Jews and the Jewish tradition?"[47] Others saw this law as a questioning of the Abrahamic religions. The National Association of Evangelicals published an announcement in the *Baltimore Sun* arguing, "Jews, Muslims, and Christians all trace our spiritual heritage back to Abraham. Biblical circumcision begins with Abraham. No American government should restrict this historic tradition. Essential religious liberties are at stake. The proposed ban violates the First Amendment's guarantee to exercise one's religious beliefs."[48] This was noteworthy because unlike Jews and Muslims, Christians are not religiously mandated to practice circumcision. As a result Governor Jerry Brown signed a bill into law that prevents California communities from banning the practice of circumcision on infant males. Assembly Bill 768, which was introduced after a San Francisco initiative on the topic of circumcision gained momentum, passed the state legislature in late August of 2011. The bill argued that anti-circumcision measures would infringe on the medical, religious and personal freedoms of parents. Sadly, the complexity of these medical, religious, and human rights questions was ignored by the legislature.

A European Praxis

The debate over legal measures that ban or allow circumcision took a different turn in Europe. According to a decision handed down by the Cologne regional court on June 26, 2012, circumcision of young boys is a criminal act, prohibited by law, even if parents have consented to the procedure.[49] The decision was grounded on the reasoning that such circumcisions cause "illegal bodily harm" to the children, and that the child's right to physical integrity supersedes parents' rights and the freedom of religion. The Jewish response was clear and immediate "Circumcision is absolutely elementary for every Jew," the organization's president, Dieter Graumann, said in an interview with the *Rheinische Post* newspaper. He warned that if the Cologne ruling were to become the legal basis for determining the legality of circumcision that "Jewish life in Germany might ultimately no longer be possible."[50] The Conference of European Rabbis called an emergency three-day meeting in Berlin to discuss what to do. Its president, Rabbi Pinchos Goldschmidt, the chief rabbi of Moscow, called the Cologne ruling the "worst attack on Jewish life since the Holocaust." Citing France's ban on Muslim veils and Switzerland's ban on the construction of new minarets for mosques, Goldschmidt suggested that the Cologne decision is part of a wider trend of intolerance against religious traditions in Europe (*Der Spiegel* 2012).

The Cologne regional court upheld the lower court's ruling, but on different grounds; that the doctor believed he was acting lawfully in the context of an unclear legal situation surrounding the practice. While the court held that religious circumcisions were illegal because they violate the child's right to physical integrity and self-determination, it differentiated such acts from instances when a circumcision is medically necessary. On December 12, 2012, in an overwhelming vote (434 to 100 votes), the German parliament voted to keep ritual circumcision legal in Germany. There were four stipulations to the law:

1. Adequate training of the practitioners for nonmedical circumcision during the first six months.
2. Does not specifically require the use of an "effective painkiller" as "according to the standards of medical practice" also covers the "necessary and effective treatment of pain in individual cases." (If no anesthesia the act remains bodily harm [Körperverletzung], but is not illegal [rechtswidrig].)

3. Parents are to be made aware of potential consequences.
4. The practice is not to be carried out by nonmedical circumcisers on children who could be at risk of complications.

However, "the ministry specifically avoids making any special provisions for circumcision for religious reasons, choosing instead to anchor it in legislation governing the rights of children to avoid requiring steps to determine the motivation of a parents' decision to have their children circumcised."[51] It is clear that the six-month window established by the law allows for most Jewish and Muslim practices to occur legally (even though Muslims can and do circumcise up to the fourteenth year of life.) What is evident is that the requirement for anesthesia violates some religious practices, and the demands for a risk assessment, as we have seen in New York City, is seen as an antireligious statement, no matter the desire of the ministry.

Why have the debates about infant male circumcision surfaced in the United States, in the UK, and in Germany (in very different forms) recently? In each instance, this certainly has to do with a contemporaneous surfacing of fierce public debates about Islam, Sharia law, and civic society in the public sphere—from the then archbishop of Canterbury, Rowan Williams, views of Sharia law in 2008 to regional attempts to outlaw these laws in American states such as Oklahoma (with virtually no Muslim community). While in the past it was the ritual practice of circumcision among Jews that was the trigger for such debates, it is now Islam. Advocates invoke the health exception, and public health authorities are placed in a position where they must either support or contradict such claims; opponents stress the violation of human rights and note the health risks. These ideological claims color the science in all directions: either blurring risk, making broader claims about efficacy, or providing rationales for the procedure. The vehemence of these debates seems in no way to be impacted by any evidence-based medical or epidemiological claims.

The health exception in the circumcision debates is analogous to the debates about the health exception in abortion: abortion is a right because women have a legal right to control of their bodies . . . unless you are opposed to abortion, in which case the rights of the fetus then trump all else. Unless (and this has recently been foregrounded in American discussions) the pregnancy is the result of rape or incest or endangers the health of the mother, the procedure is contraindicated on religious grounds. The most radical opponents to abortion dismiss the first two exceptions, but the health exception seems always to remain, even among those most opposed to the procedure. In the modern world, the health exception—argued on both sides of the circumcision debate—can in truth never be resolved, in regard to abortion or to circumcision. One observer's health risk is another's valid intervention; one observer's sense of the rights of any category may or may not be trumped by the health risk.

Over and over again, the health exception is used to argue for or against what is in its essence a religious practice. One could see in this a justification for advocating or for banning this practice if the use of science was autonomous. But in every case, including the most recent public health advocacy, there is the assumption that there is an essential relationship between circumcision and health even though what is defined as health is constantly shifting. James Boon stressed that circumcision is first and foremost a cultural practice that is given meaning by its contrasting the bodies that are marked by the practice from those that are not. Thus the qualities ascribed to such a contrast, beauty or ugliness, health or mutilation, belonging or being excluded, are available for other contexts such as medicine in which they are given scientific readings depending whether one is an advocate or an opponent of the practice. With the debates about the health exception it is clear that one of the cultures that reads circumcision is that of medicine, as its adversarial position for or against simply reflects again Boon's claim of its function "separating an 'us' from a 'them' [as] entangled in various discourses of identity and distancing."

Notes

1. James A. Boon. "Circumscribing Circumcision/Uncircumcision: An Essay amidst the History of Difficult Description." In Stuart B. Schwartz, ed. *Implicit Understandings.* (Cambridge: Cambridge University Press, 1994), 556–85, here 556. See also James Boon. *Other Tribes, Other Scribes.* (New York: Cambridge University Press, 1982), 162–68; *Affinities and Extremes.* (Chicago: University of Chicago Press, 1990), 55–60; *Verging on Extra-vagance.* (Princeton, N.J.: Princeton University Press, 1999), See 43–47, where he contrasts Montaigne and the nineteenth-century American commentator P. C. Remondino's views.
2. On the history and culture of circumcision see S. J. Waszak. "The Historic Significance of Circumcision." *Obstetrics and Gynecology* 51 (1978): 499–501; E. Grossman and N. A. Posner. "Surgical Circumcision of Neonates: A History of its Development." *Obstetrics and Gynecology* 58 (1981): 241–46; Elliot A. Grossman. *Circumcision: A Pictorial Atlas of its History, Instrument Development and Operative Techniques.* (Great Neck, NY: Todd & Honeywell, 1982); John J. Collins. "A Symbol of Otherness: Circumcision and Salvation in the First Century." In Jacob Neusner and Ernest S. Frerichs, eds. *"To See*

Ourselves as Others See Us": Christians, Jews, "Others," in Late Antiquity. (Chico, CA: Scholars Press, 1985), 163–85; Desmond Morris. *Bodywatching.* (London: Jonathan Cape, 1985), 218–20; Claude Lévi-Strauss. "Exode sur Exode." *Homme* 28(1988): 106–7; Nigel Allan. "A Polish Rabbi's Circumcision Manual." *Medical History* 33(1989): 2 47–54; Moisés Trachtenberg and Philip Slotkin. "Circumcision, Crucifixion, and AntiSemitism: The Antithetical Character of Ideologies and Their Symbol Which Contain Crossed Lines." *International Review of Psycho-Analysis* 16 (1989): 459–71; Howard Eilberg-Schwartz. 1990. *The Savage in Judaism: An Anthropology of Israelite Religion and Ancient Judaism.* Bloomington: Indiana University Press. 141–76; Moisés Trachtenberg. 1990. *Psicanálise da circuncisâo.* Porto Alegre: Sagra; Malek Chebel. 1992. *Histoire de la circoncision: des origines a nos jours.* Paris: Balland; Howard Eilberg-Schwartz. 1994. *God's Phallus and Other Problems for Men in Monotheism.* Boston: Beacon; David Gollaher. 2000. *Circumcision: A History of the World's Most Controversial Surgery.* New York: Basic Books; Elizabeth Wyner Mark. 2003. *The Covenant of Circumcision: New Perspectives on an Ancient Jewish Rite.* Hanover, NH: Brandeis University Press, published by University Press of New England, 2003); Shaye J. D. Cohen. 2005. *Why Aren't Jewish Women Circumcised? Gender And Covenant In Judaism.* Berkeley: University of California Press; Eric Kline Silverman. 2006. *From Abraham to America. A History of Jewish Circumcision.* Lanham, MD: Rowman & Littlefield Publishers; Robin Judd. 2007. *Contested Rituals: Circumcision, Kosher Butchering, and Jewish Political Life in Germany, 1843–1933.* Ithaca: Cornell University Press. Recently, I have provided a long comment on Marie Fox and Michael Thomson Fox. 2012. "The New Politics of Male Circumcision: HIV/AIDS, Health Law and Social Justice." *Legal Studies* 32: 255–281 *in Global Discourse: An Interdisciplinary Journal of Current Affairs and Applied Contemporary Thought* 3: 2 (2013): 376–378.

3. Daniel M. Harrison, "Rethinking Circumcision and Sexuality in the United States," *Sexualities* 5(2002): 300–316.
4. American Academy of Pediatrics. 1971. *American Academy of Pediatrics Committee on Fetus and Newborn, Standards And Recommendation For Hospital Care Of Newborn Infants.* Accessed at http://www.cirp.org/library/statements/aap/#1971 on September 14, 2013.
5. American Academy of Pediatrics. 1999. "American Academy of Pediatrics Task Force on Circumcision, Circumcision Policy Statement." *Pediatrics* 103(3): 686, 686. Accessed at *http://pediatrics.aappublications.org/content/103/3/686.full* on September 14, 2013.
6. American Academy of Pediatrics. 2012. "Circumcision Policy Statement: Task Force on Circumcision." *Pediatrics* 130(3): 585–586. Accessed from http://pediatrics.aappublications.org/content/103/3/686.short on September 12, 2013.
7. Deutsche Akademie für Kinder-und Jugendmedizin. 2012. "Stellungnahme zur Beschneidung von minderjährigen Jungen Kommission für ethische Fragen der DAKJ." Accessed from http://dakj.de/media/stellungnahmen/ethische-fragen/2012_Stellungnahme_Beschneidung.pdf on September 12, 2013.
8. As reflected in the title of the major book of 1896 by Andrew Dickson White, *A History of the Warfare of Science with Theology in Christendom.* New York: D. Appelton, 1896.

9. Sander L. Gilman. "Barbaric' Rituals?" In Joshua Cohen, Matthew Howard, and Martha C. Nussbaum, eds. *Is Multiculturalism Bad for Women?* (Princeton: Princeton University Press, 1999), 53–58. Male circumcision is so often treated in the West as acceptable (with the exception of practices like subincision in Oceania) while female circumcision is not, as if the only real equivalent to female circumcision is a penectomy? Kirsten Bell actually uses this question to trace the debates on the health benefits of male circumcision (see Kirsten Bell, "Genital Cutting and Western Discourses on Sexuality." *MAQ* 19:2 (2005): 125-48). On female genital cutting see the special edition edited by Richard Schweder, ed. *The End of Tolerance: Engaging Cultural Differences. Daedalus* 129, No. 4, (Fall, 2000).
10. Rachel Dann, ed. *Current Research in Egyptology 2004: Proceedings of the Fifth Annual Symposium which took place at the University of Durham, January 2004.* (Oxford: Oxbow Books, 2006), p. 73.
11. William Arrowsmith, trans. *The Satyricon of Petronius.* (Ann Arbor: University of Michigan Press, 1959), p. 102.4.
12. Tacitus. *The Histories.* Books IV–V. In Clifford H. Moore, trans. *Tacitus in Five Volumes III: The Histories, Book IV–V. The Annals, Books I-III.* (Cambridge, Mass.: Harvard University Press, 1969), p. 5.5.
13. F. Marx. Celsus. *De medicina.* Vol 1. In W. C. Spencer, trans. *Corpus Medicorum Latinorum,* Loeb Classical Library. (Cambridge, MA: Harvard University Press, 1938), p. 118.
14. Jody P. Rubin. "Celsus's Decircumcision Operation: Medical And Historical Implication." *Urology* 16 (1980): 121–124.
15. William Whiston, trans. *Works of Josephus: Antiquities of the Jews.* (Philadelphia: The John C. Winston Company, 1954), p. 256.
16. Peder Borgen. *Philo: An Exegete for His Time.* (Leiden: Brill, 1997), here, p. 159.
17. Cited by Boon, *Other Scribes,* (1982, here p. 29); I have corrected the translation to reflect the comments by Shaya Cohen, p. 230.
18. Benedikt de Spinoza. *A Theologico-Political Treatise and Political Treatise.* (New York: Dover, 1951), p. 15.
19. James A. Boon. *The Anthropological Romance of Bali, 1597–1972: Dynamic Perspectives in Marriage and Caste, Politics and Religion.* (Cambridge: Cambridge University Press, 1977), p. 212.
20. Immanuel Kant. "Religion within the Boundaries of Mere Reason." In Allan Wood, trans. *Religion and Rational Theology.* (Cambridge: Cambridge University Press, 1996), pp. 155–156.
21. Paolo Mantegazza. *The Sexual Relations of Mankind.* Victor Robinson, trans. (New York: Eugenics Pub. Co., 1935), p. 99.
22. Johann David Michaelis. *Orientalische und Exegetische Bibliothek.* (Frankfurt am Main: Johann Gottlieb Garbe, 1773), p. 94.
23. Johann Friedrich Blumenbach. *Über den Bildungstrieb und das Zeugungsgeschäfte.* L. v. Kàrolyi, ed. (Stuttgart: Gustav Fischer, 1971), p. 69.
24. Schiller, Friedrich. *Werke.* Vol. 3. Weimar: (Hermann Böhlaus Nachfolger, 1943), p. 22.
25. On Schiller and the Jews see Norbert Oellers. "Goethe und Schiller in ihrem Verhältnis zum Judentum." In Hans Otto Horch and Horst Denkler, eds. *Conditio Judaica: Judentum, Antisemitismus und deutschsprachgige Literatur vom 18. Jahrhundert bis zum ersten* (Weltkrieg. Tübingen: Niemeyer, 1988), 108–130.

26. Charles Darwin. *The Variation of Animals and Plants under Domestication*. Vol. 2. (London: John Murray, 1868), p. 23.
27. "Reports of Societies from June." 5 June 1920. *British Medical Journal*. 1(3103): 768.
28. Leopold Zunz. *Gutachten über die Beschneidung*. (Frankfurt am Main: J. F. Bach, 1844); Lawrence A Hoffman. *Covenant of Blood: Circumcision and Gender in Rabbinic Judaism*. (Chicago: University of Chicago Press, 1996); Jacob Katz. "The Controversy over the *Mezizah*: The Unrestricted Execution of the Rite of Circumcision" and "The Struggle over Preserving the Rite of Circumcision in the First Part of the Nineteenth Century." In his *Divine Law in Human Hands: Case Studies in Halakhic Flexibility*. (Jerusalem: Magnes Press, 1998), pp. 320–402.
29. Anonymous. "Die rituelle Beschneidung bei den Juden und ihre Gefahren." *Journal für Kinderkrankheiten* 59(1872): 367–72.
30. Peter Charles Remondino. *History of Circumcision from the Earliest Times to the Present*. (Philadelphia: F. A. Davis, 1891), p. 66.
31. Johann Friedrich Dieffenbach. *Die operative Chirugie*. Vol. 1. (Leipzig: F. A. Brockhaus, 1845). 515–22, here p. 517.
32. John S. Billings, "Vital Statistics of the Jews." *North American Review* 153(1891): 70–84, here p. 70.
33. Robert Fowler. "What are the Effects of Circumcision?" *The Lancet* 75.1911(1860): 382.
34. Robert Darby. *A Surgical Temptation: The Demonization of the Foreskin and the Rise of Circumcision in Britain*. (Chicago: University of Chicago Press, 2005), here p. 260.
35. Marina Gilman, Sander Gilman, and Michael M. Johns. "Human Papillomavirus, Abstinence, and the Other Risks." *The Lancet* 373.9673 (2009): 1420–1421.
36. E. J. Schoen, "Ode to the Circumcised Male." *American Journal of Disease of Childhood* 141 (1987): 128.
37. Johanna Schiratzki. "Banning God's Law In The Name Of The Holy Body - The Nordic Position On Ritual Male Circumcision." *The Family in Law* 5 (2011): 35–53.
38. D.M. Gairdner. "The Fate of the Foreskin: A Study of Circumcision." *British Medical Journal* 2(1949): 1433–7.
39. See Johanna Schiratzki. *Best Interests of the Child*. Oxford Bibliographies in Childhood Studies. Heather Montgomery, ed. New York: Oxford University Press, 2013).
40. *Rotterdams Dagblad*. "Hirsi Ali wil verbod besnijdenis jongens." *Rotterdams Dagblad* (4 October 2004).
41. Sharon Otterman. "Board Votes to Regulate Circumcision, Citing Risks." *The New York Times Online*. (13 September 2012). Accessed at http://www.nytimes.com/2012/09/14/nyregion/health-board-votes-to-regulate-jewish-circumcision-ritual.html on September 13 2013.
42. Susan Bewley, and Sarah Strandjord. "Letters." *Pediatrics* 130.3 (2012): 585–586.
43. Muhammad Lufti Al-Sabbagh. "Islamic Ruling on Male and Female Circumcision." (1996) In The World Health Organization Eastern Mediterranean. *The Right Path to Health: Health Education and Religion*. Accessed

at http://www.emro.who.int/vip/PDF/female_male_circumcision_en.pdf on September 14, 2013.

44. Gregory J. Boyle, and George Hill. "Sub-Saharan African Randomised Clinical Trials into Male Circumcision and HIV Transmission: Methodological, Ethical and Legal Concerns." *Journal of Law and Medicine* 19.2 (2011): 316–34, here p. 316.

45. Morten Frisch, *et al.* "Commentary: Cultural Bias in the AAP's 2012 Technical Report and Policy Statement on Male Circumcision." *Pediatrics* (Published Online March 18, 2013). Accessed at http://pediatrics.aappublications.org/content/early/2013/03/12/peds.2012-2896 on September 15, 2013.

46. S. C. Kalichman, L. Eaton, and S. D. Pinkerton. "Male Circumcision in HIV Prevention. *The Lancet* 369(2007): 1597–1599; S. R. Sawires, S. L. Dworkin, A. Fiamma, D. Peacock, and G. Szekeres, et al. "Male Circumcision and HIV/AIDS: Challenges and Opportunities." *The Lancet* 369(2007): 708–71; S. C. Kalichman, "Neonatal Circumcision for HIV Prevention: Cost, Culture, and Behavioral Considerations." PLoS Med 7.1 (2010): e1000219.

47. David Wolpe. "Circumcision Ban Another Attack on Judaism." *The Washington Post Online.* (6 June 2011). Accessed at http://www.washingtonpost.com/blogs/on-faith/post/circumcision-ban-another-attack-on-judaism/2011/06/06/AGloVJKH_blog.html on September 15, 2013.

48. Brown, Matthew Hay. "Evangelicals Join Jews Against Circumcision Ban." *The Baltimore Sun Online.* (9 June 2011). Accessed at http://weblogs.baltimoresun.com/news/faith/christianity/ on September 12, 2013.

49. Press Release, Landesgericht Köln, Urteile des Amtsgerichts und des Landgerichts Köln zur Strafbarkeit von Beschneidungen nicht einwilligungsfähiger Jungen aus rein religiösen Gründe [Judgments of the Local District Court and of the Cologne Regional Court on the Criminalization of Circumcision of Non-Consensual Boys for Purely Religious Reasons], JUSTIZ-ONLINE [Landgericht Köln website] (June 26, 2012); Decision of May 7, 2012 [in German], Docket No. Az. 151 Ns 169/11, Landgericht Köln Cologne.) http://www.loc.gov/lawweb/servlet/lloc_news?disp3_1205403226_text Accessed on September 14, 2012.

50. *Der Spiegel.* "The World from Berlin: Circumcision Ruling Is 'a Shameful Farce for Germany.'" *Der Spiegel Online.* (12 July 2012). Accessed at http://www.spiegel.de/international/germany/german-press-review-on-outlash-against-court-s-circumcision-ruling-a-844271.html on September 15, 2013.

51. Melissa Eddy. "Proposal Sets Circumcision Regulations in Germany." *The New York Times Online.* (26 September 2012). Accessed at http://www.nytimes.com/2012/09/27/world/europe/27iht-circumcision27.html on September 15, 2012.

Questions

How can the history of religion and the history of health intersect?

Why are the sexual organs of particular importance in the intersection of religion and health in the West?

Why does Christianity abandon infant male circumcision?

How do question of infection play a role in the debates about allowing or forbidding circumcision?

Are there other cases of religious objection to or advocacy of interventions preventing infection?

What are the "human rights" involved in the debate about circumcision?

Case Two

Face Transplants: Authentic Faces?

Problems: Do our faces reflect who we are, who we want to be, or who our societies want us to be? What is the difference between enhancement and reconstruction? How do cultural assumptions concerning what makes our appearance "authentic" underlie the definition of each concept? In this chapter, we will explore the claim that face transplants reconstruct the face while aesthetic surgery enhances the way we want to look. Our case studies spans the history of the nose job in nineteenth-century Berlin to face transplants in the twenty-first century—and a look at the meanings ascribed to Michael Jackson's face following his death.

Bodies and Authenticity

The idea that there is an "authentic" body and face is a cultural truism, contradicted by the simple realization that most cultures permit or indeed require our bodies to be altered. Tattooing, scarification, and (as we have already read) circumcision, are all forms of body modification with religious and secular dimensions. Likewise, what we see as modern surgical or medical interventions that open and alter the body appear to have been widely practiced, even though some forms, such as early forms of trepanning (opening the skull) may indeed have had more of a religious than a medical basis. Certainly the modern history of reconstructive and aesthetic surgery in restoring or improving the body and the face is an area where very hard questions have been asked as to whether such interventions violate either religious claims calling for an acceptance of the body given to you by God or social claims criticizing vanity passing itself off as medicine.[1] And yet our society undertakes such bodily alterations regularly whether it is in public health requirements for vaccination against disease or the fashion of ear piercing.

We have a body that is constantly changing—through developmental processes such as aging as well as through a wide range of culturally required or permitted interventions. We however are constantly debating the nature, definition, or scope of what constitutes an "authentic body" as if the body were static and unchanging. Authenticity itself is described by Michael H. Krenis and Brian M. Goldman as a concept

> at the "limits of language," being loosely described in such diverse topics as ethics, well-being, consciousness, subjectivity, self-processes, and social or relational contexts, or characterized in terms of its opposite (i.e., inauthenticity), with references to inauthentic living, false-self behaviors, or self-deception.[2]

Bodily authenticity is thus very much in the eye of the beholder. Understanding this does not vitiate the need to parse what the persistent anxiety about the "inauthentic" body represents.

The notion that one has a God-given or natural (and therefore authentic) body becomes one of the truisms in the debates about the rise of modern aesthetic surgery in the late nineteenth century. Men were the initial patrons of aesthetic interventions in the 1890s; only by the 1920s is aesthetic surgery seen as something undertaken primarily by women. Yet from their infancy, such procedures were understood both by patients and their surgeons as a means of producing the faces they both desire. These desired faces were authentic faces because of the standards for appearance more in keeping with that demanded by the society in which doctor and patient lived; but were simultaneously labeled as the products of "vanity," that is, as "inauthentic." As a journalist recently opined concerning cosmetic surgery:

> "It's vain and shallow. It's a sign of decadence and the decline of Western civilization," I lamented. "It's not natural and authentic. . . . I want my face to be a record of who I am, where I've been, what I've been through, a visual memoir of my life and times. Cosmetic surgery turns it into a work of fiction."[3]

Most of the surgical interventions that were labeled inauthentic by early critics of aesthetic surgery involved the face: facelifts, eyelid lifts, ear tucks, and certainly the most popular aesthetic intervention of the first age of modern aesthetic surgery, the nose job.[4]

Authentic Noses

It was in the 1890s that the most notable of German Jewish aesthetic surgeons, Jacques Joseph (1865–1934), developed a series of procedures to alter the shape of the Jewish face in Wilhelminian Germany. Equally importantly, he was the first to advance an explanation that for such alterations based on their psychological effectiveness rather than solely on their somatic success. He created a new sense of "authenticity" in claiming that the happiness resulting from his surgeries made more content and therefore more authentic patients.

Jacques Joseph (1865–1934) was born Jakob Joseph; he had altered his "too-Jewish" name when he studied medicine in Berlin and Leipzig. He was being trained as an orthopedic surgeon under Julius Wolff (1836–1902), one of the leaders in that field. Wolff established the "law of the transformation of the skeleton," which argued that every function of the skeleton could be described through the laws of mechanics and that any change in the relationship between single components of the skeleton would lead to a functional and physiological change of the external form of the entire skeleton.[5] Orthopedics, more than any other medical specialty of the period, presented the challenge of altering the visible errors of development so as to restore a "normal" function. Wolff's view was that all such alterations had solely functional and structural meanings.

Even though the flat feet attributed to the Jews were another sign of Jewish inferiority, Joseph's interests did not lie with the foot, but elsewhere in the anatomy. In 1896, he undertook a corrective procedure on a young child with protruding ears. According to the child's mother, the boy had suffered from humiliation in school because of his appearance. Rather than correcting his appearance, it was, first and foremost, the child's unhappiness with being different that Joseph was correcting. Abnormally big and protruding ears alone might account for the child's unhappiness. But it was the specific cultural meaning of protruding ears at the close of the nineteenth century that really added insult to injury. Such ears were a sign of social stigma in Joseph's Berlin. The racial anthropologist Hans Günther summarizes the turn-of-the-century view that Jews, especially males, have "fleshy ear lobes" and "large, red ears" more frequently than other peoples do. They have "prominent ears that stick out." According to Günther, prominent ears are especially prevalent among "Jewish children; one refers to them in Austria as 'Moritz ears.'"[6] Moritz (Morris) was a typical Jewish name of the day. They are the "elongated ears" which appear as the "ill-shapen ears of great size like those of a bat," according to an English-language anti-Semitic text of 1888.[7]

The procedure to change the appearance of the child's protruding ears was successful, and he was freed of his visible stigma. But remember that Wolff had stressed the functional changes that such procedures accomplished. In Berlin in the 1890s this sort of operation was seen as "beauty" surgery rather than "real" surgery. Wolff promptly dismissed Joseph as his assistant. When Joseph was dismissed, Wolff told him that one simply did not undertake surgical procedures for vanity's sake. A child's protruding ears were not in the same class as a functional disability, such as a club foot, nor did it present the same pressing need for a solution as cases requiring the reconstruction of the external ear, which had been a major problem for surgeons from the earliest written accounts.[8] (The congenital absence of the external ear [microtia] was often attributed to hereditary syphilis. This would have been grounds to operate!)

After being dismissed from Wolff's clinic, Joseph opened a private surgical practice in Berlin. In January 1898, a twenty-eight-year-old man came to him, having heard of the successful operation on the child's ears. He complained that

> his nose was the source of considerable annoyance. Wherever he went, everybody stared at him; often, he was the target of remarks or ridiculing gestures. On account of this he became melancholic, withdrew almost completely from social life, and had the earnest desire to be relieved of this deformity.[9]

The symptoms were analogous to those of the young boy whose ears Joseph had repaired.

Joseph took the young man's case and proceeded to perform his first reduction rhinoplasty, cutting through the skin of the nose to reduce its size and alter its shape by chipping away the bone and removing the cartilage. On May 11, 1898, he reported on this operation before the Berlin Medical Society. In that report, Joseph provided a detailed "scientific" rationale for performing a medical procedure on an otherwise completely healthy individual:

> The psychological effect of the operation is of utmost importance. The depressed attitude of the patient subsided completely. He is happy to move around unnoticed. His happiness in life has increased, his wife

> was glad to report; the patient who formerly avoided social contact now wishes to attend and give parties. In other words, he is happy over the results.[10]

The patient no longer felt himself marked by the form of his nose. He was cured of the "disease" of "nostrility." In his own eyes, he looked less different from the group he desired to join—the non-Jews. Joseph had undertaken a surgical procedure, which had cured his patient's psychological disorder! Yet he had left scars, which pointed

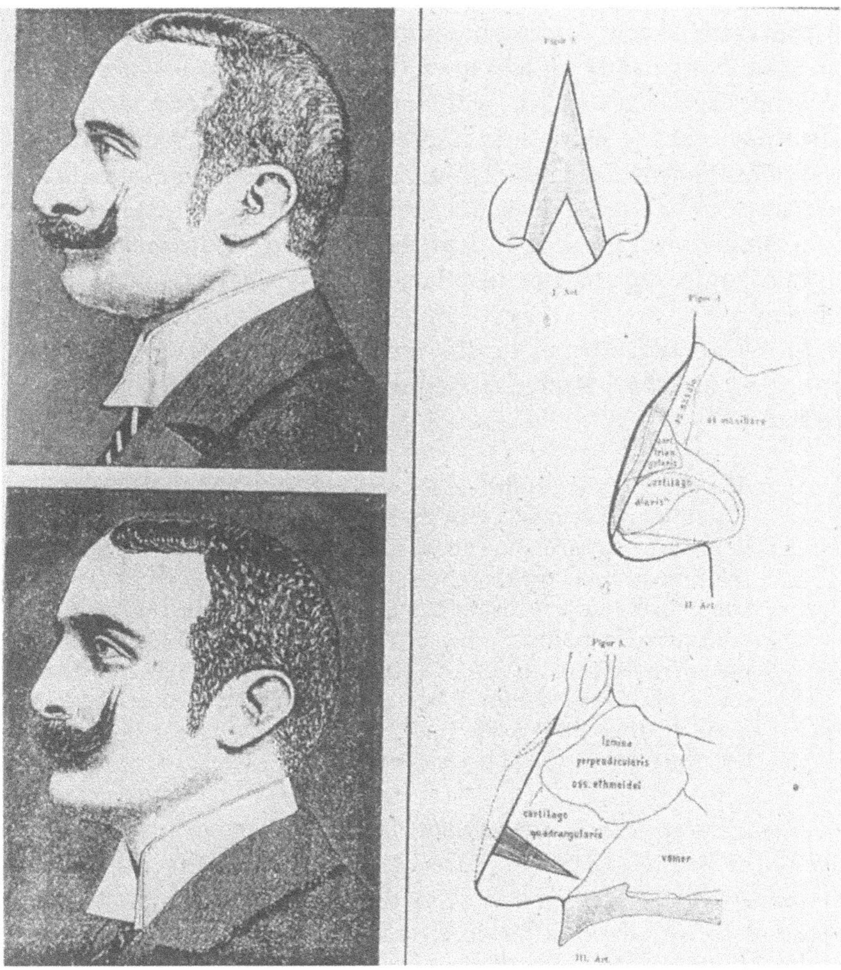

Figure 2.1. The first, modern nasal reduction, from Jacques Joseph's "Über die operative Verkleinerung einer Nase (Rhinomiosis)." *Berliner klinische Wochenschrift* 40 (1898): 882-85.

to the procedure itself, and this became a major concern of Joseph's. He warned his colleagues that "disclosure to the patient on the problem of scarring is very important. Many patients, however, will consider even simple scars too conspicuous. . . ."[11] He raised the specter of a court case in which the "unsightly scar might represent a greater degree of disfigurement than the enlarged cartilage [of the nose] presented previously."[12] More centrally though, surgical scars, unlike dueling scars, reveal the inauthencity of the body and the effort to pass through medical intervention.

On April 19, 1904, Joseph undertook his removal of a hump from within the nose using cartilaginous incisions. He retrospectively commented that in 1898 he had used the extranasal procedure, which "caused a scar, but this scar will be hardly visible after a short time, assuming that the incision is sutured exactly."[13] But "hardly visible" was not sufficient. Even the slightest scar was enough to evoke a visual memory of the too-big nose. The invisibility of the patient hinged on the elimination of the scar. Both patients needed to become (in)visible to pass. And Joseph had learned that only (in)visibility left his patients "happy."

In his summary paper on the reduction of the size of the nose published in 1904, Joseph commented on the psychology of his male patients:

> The patients were embarrassed and self-conscious in their dealings with their fellow men, often shy and unsociable, and had the urgent desire to become free and unconstrained. Several complained of sensitive drawbacks in the exercise of their profession. As executives they could hardly enforce their authority; in their business connections (as salesmen, for example), they often suffered material losses. . . . The operative nasal reduction—this is my firm conviction—will also in the future restore the joy of living to many a wretched creature and, if his deformity has been hindering him in his career, it will allow him the full exercise of his aptitudes.[14]

According to Joseph, the patient "is happy to move around unnoticed." The visibility of the Jew (often defined in the nineteenth century in terms of his mercantile ability) made it impossible for him to compete equally with the non-Jew in the economic world at the turn of the century. Only vanishing into the visual norm and passing as non-Jewish in terms of his appearance enabled the young Jewish male to become part of the general society.

Now this intervention quickly becomes a broadly used practice in Central Europe. The new authenticity is immediately challenged as "inauthentic." Thus one of the best known and most widely read columnists for the major daily newspaper the *New Free Press* in Vienna writes a *Feuilleton* entitled "New Noses" in 1903.

> It is now a question of style. . . . [E]very province must have its own nose! Still others will let national interests rather than the lottery of birth determine the selection of the nose. Whatever the case, even in this matter we will certainly see the reappearance of the demand that those closest as well as most distant be converted to a specific nasal shape, instead of each being happy with the cut of his/her nose.[15] ["statt jeden nach seiner Façon sich schnäuzen zu lassen"]

Theodor Herzl was mocking the claims of the new surgery and also commenting on the claim that a new authenticity could be achieved by Jews through the means of physically vanishing into European society. Herzl founded modern Zionism at more or less the same moment that Joseph was developing modern aesthetic surgery. He demanded that Jews be recognized as an authentic nation, not merely as Jewish citizens of a European state. His ironic *pointe* is made in the final line of the quote; he parodies the Enlightenment comment by Friedrich II of Prussia on religious freedom, who said "that each should become happy after their own manner." Now, according to Herzl's sarcastic observation, it is that each should become happy through the acquisition of a new nose. Such a belief in physical transformation leaves one with an inauthentic nose.

Authentic Faces Anew?

The image of an inauthentic face seems more or less appropriate as a symbol for aesthetic procedures given our contemporary anxiety about vanity. Vanity is understood as a desire for inherently something inauthentic. Yet the now almost universal acceptance by most corners of Western society of aesthetic interventions seems also to argue that such faces are deemed more and more acceptable if not more authentic than their "natural" visage by larger and larger numbers of patients. The same confusion over what constitutes (in)authenticity arose with the first face allotransplant in 2005 a team in Amiens, France, conducted by the facio-maxillary surgeon Bernard Devauchelle as part of the team under lead surgeon Joan Pere Barret. The patient, Isabelle Dinoire, received her partial face transplant in December of that year.[16] The public response was immediate and questioning: was this new face really "her" face or was it the cadaver's face? Or a mix of both? Was it a "real" face or merely a hybrid? The rumor that the source of the face had committed suicide lead to the speculation that the transplant would have ". . . implications for Ms. Dinoire's future, because if true, and if the transplant is successful, it would mean that for the rest of her life, she would see in the mirror the nose, mouth and chin of a woman who herself met a brutal end."[17] There may well have been some question of whether Dinoire was receiving a face that had suffered organ damage had it come from someone who died of a suicide by hanging, as Devauchelle stated at the time, but the idea that she would be looking at someone else's face after the procedure evokes immediately the idea that the face is not really the patient's own, but rather a simulacrum, a virtual but inauthentic face.[18]

The line between authentic and inauthentic faces was not lost on the Amien team. For Devauchelle, the challenge was a surgical one, not an epistemological one, as he stated in a later interview:

> "What does a face mean?" he said. "Be careful. Lots of philosophers and artists speak and write of the significance of the face. It is provocative, but I am not sure. For me, the face is exactly like an organ. It is no more, no less. There is the heart, liver, brain-and the face. Everyone is looking for truth in the face. For a surgeon, it is skin, tissue, muscle, blood."[19]

Yet there seems always to be the question of what makes a transplanted face real to the patient and real to the world in which the patient

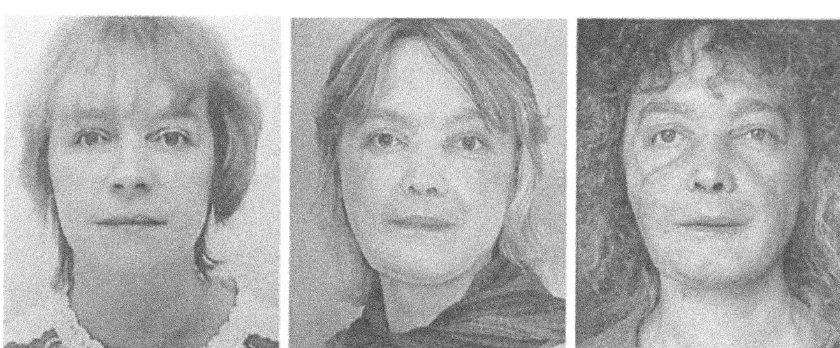

Figure 2.2. Left to right: Dinoire before the dog attack; one year after the transplant surgery with makeup; and six months later without makeup. Image credits: dailymail.co.uk.

lives. In Devauchelle's account, the authenticity of the face is based on the anonymity of its biological properties.

In my conversation with Bernard Devauchelle at the Transplantation conference at Cerisy in May 2012 it was clear that he (and all subsequent face transplant surgeons) had a sense of what would make someone an unacceptable (or "inauthentic") donor. Clearly he said the gender had to be the same, and the skin color also: no male face on a female patient and no black face on a white patient. Indeed, he noted that subsequent to the Denoire transplant, there was at least one case where he rejected a potential donor as inappropriate. The donor face was not technically inappropriate but aesthetically inappropriate—and that in the light of the rather rare occurrence of such donors.[20] Can one imagine a hybrid face, part male, part female, part white, part black, part aged, part youthful? Of course, one can, but such a face would signal (at least at the moment) its cultural inauthenticity. Devauchelle had confronted at least one such question earlier, as he explained in an interview: "Devauchelle . . . told me that a woman had come to see him with her daughter, who had a traumatic facial injury. 'The mother said, "I want to give my face to my daughter,"' he told me. 'And I had to explain—.' He took a drag, exhaled, and shook his head. 'It is quite a burden,' he said."[21] Clearly, no living donors would be allowed, no matter how altruistic their claims nor how much they look like the patient.

The fantasy of the face transplant is that one now has the visage of a dead person and that one becomes, in an unstated way, that person.[22] Your face is you; if you have another person's face you are that person. Even before the first transplant was undertaken, this question was raised:

> Appearance is dictated not just by skin, but by bone structure, and surgeons are not sure how closely a reconstructed face would resemble a donor's at the end of the operation. The technical challenges are huge. So are the ethical dilemmas. "The main problem in these people is coming to terms with their new appearance. And they'd have to come to terms with a new appearance anyway. So why are you doing it?" said Peter Rowe, the chairman of the ethical committee of the British Transplantation Society.[23]

Is the new face an authentic one? That is, as Jacques Joseph queried in regard to his patients, is the patient able to be happy with this new state? Or is it inauthentic, in that the transplant patient is haunted by the face of another person and therefore cannot be happy?

After the first transplant was actually undertaken by the surgeons in Amiens the question became pointed:

> In some ineffable way, though, a person's face is the person, inseparable from her external identity and her sense of self. As Ralph Waldo Emerson wrote: "A man finds room in the few square inches of the face for the traits of all his ancestors; for the expression of all his history, and his wants."[24]

Your face is who you are, more than another part of you:

> The face has always been central to a person's identity. It's how we think of each other, how we reflect emotion and pain, and its primacy is reflected in our language. We "face the music" or "put our best face forward." When your reputation is damaged, you have "lost face." In other words, how you look is not simply a matter of vanity.[25]

It is who you are.

This view of the face as the most important marker of self is precisely the same problem raised by Herzl a century before. Can you be yourself (whatever that means) when you have someone else's face or nose? In the history of transplants we did see this claim about authenticity before. When Christiaan Barnard performed the world's first human heart transplant operation on December 3, 1967, the question was raised immediately: if you have someone else's heart do you have their emotions, their soul? Now the "heart" here was functioning as a metaphor.[26] Medicine, at least, assumed that the heart was a muscle, not a surrogate for the soul. Popular opinion believed that the heart was where our soul rested, acting as sort of surrogate for the essence of what makes a human being human. This view has not vanished, even in an age where heart transplants have become medically commonplace.

> The progress of medical science in the past 30 years has been so rapid that yesterday's miracles are tomorrow's commonplace procedures. So it has proved with heart transplants, which have become almost routine in hospitals around the world.... [D]onor patients could not only be acquiring the organs but also the memories—or even the soul—of the donor.

A case study seemed to confirm this: A young man is reported to have written

> haunting lyrics, the boy sang about how he felt destined to die and donate his heart. After his death, his heart was transplanted into an

> 18-year-old girl named Danielle. When the boy's parents met Danielle, they played some of his music and she, despite never having heard the song before, knew the words and was able to complete the lyrics.[27]

This account is tabloid journalism, based on questionable scientific research by Gary E. Schwartz, PhD, director of the VERITAS Research Program, professor of psychology, medicine, neurology, psychiatry, and surgery at the University of Arizona. However, the power of the heart as the organ of the soul still seems to haunt tabloid notions of the authenticity of heart transplantation.

No one would seriously make this claim about kidneys or livers (not even in France, which has a special cultural reading of "*ma foie*," "my liver" as one of the popular sources of many ailments) or corneas or bone marrow. Does a cornea transplant patient see the world through the eyes of the cadaver from which the corneas were taken?[28] Hearts and faces seem to have meanings that are more highly charged than opposed to other aspects of the body. The transplantation of these organs seems not to be able to be completely routinized over time.[29] The twenty-third face allotransplant patient was Richard Lee Norris. His procedure occurred on March 19–20, 2012, at the University of Maryland Medical Center in the United States. The surgical team performed the most extensive full face transplant to date, replacing everything from the hairline to the collarbone, including the upper and lower jawbones, teeth, and a portion of the tongue. The popular response remained much the same:

> The "after" photo, taken just six days following the 36-hour surgery, shows—in striking contrast to his tragically misshapen "in-between" face—a regular, rather unremarkable male visage that will only improve as it fully heals. Richard Lee Norris should find many reasons to smile from now on. YET WHILE rejoicing at this man's passage from nightmare to normality, I couldn't help wondering about the reality of living with a face that (a) once belonged to someone else, and (b) bears little or no resemblance to the one he originally had. Though Norris must feel delivered from a fate worse than death, there is something surreal and unnerving about it, like a page out of science fiction come alive. Is this transformed Norris simply the old Norris in a new wrapping, as it were, or will his new face affect everything that lies behind it? Might he have exchanged one mask for another? "It's a blend of two individuals," Dr. Eduardo Rodriguez, who led the surgical team of more than 100 medical professionals, told reporters. "But behind the soft tissue, behind the skeleton—it's Richard."[30]

That the question of identity is raised is important. The key to the problem is the notion of a cadaver transplant. Comparing the popular response to transplants from cadavers to the response to face reattachments—the restoration of the "original" face—helps to reveal the origins of our discomfort/suspicion of the face transplant.

When the full-face replant procedure was undertaken in 1994 on a nine year-old girl whose face was ripped off when her hair was caught in a thresher, there was no claim of a "new soul," only reports of the technical prowess of the doctors in reattaching the face and scalp.[31]

> . . . Sandeep Kauer, a nine-year-old Punjabi girl whose face and scalp were ripped off by a grass-cutting machine. . . . [T]he most horrifying thing was a photograph of her disembodied face, which looked like a discarded part of a doll. The local doctor drove Sandeep—still conscious—three hours on his scooter to the nearest emergency ward, her face in a plastic bag. An expert micro-surgeon happened to be on duty, and decided to try the world's first full-face reattachment. Ten years on, Sandeep had deep scarring, but looked pretty good.[32]

In other cases of reattachment prior to 2005, it was the technical expertise that was the focus of attention:

> While three decades of research has meant that reattachment of body parts is considered routine, there are still cases that astound the doctors. The woman whose face and scalp was severed was one.
>
> She was flown to St Vincent's from Shepparton by air ambulance.
>
> Professor Morrison, who headed the team that day, says reattaching scalps is a common procedure. "When the woman came in her head was covered in bloody bandages and the scalp was in a separate container (on ice)," he says. "Then I unwrapped the scalp and there was a face staring at me."
>
> . . . The tissue of the face had been ripped off close to the surface where the blood vessels branch off into thread-like capillaries. Each artery and vein had to be tagged and the ends attached to grafts made from veins elsewhere on her body. Damaged vessels can't be joined - they must be cleanly cut - which often leaves them short. Vein grafts can make up the distance needed to join the two ends.[33]

There is no question here of a "character transplantation." The only question is whether doctors have the technical ability to undertake such a complex procedure. In the end, patients who undergoes a facial reattachment are their original self, because your face is your face.

Character Transplantations?

Are you more than your face? Or is the question of your very essence tied to your appearance? Certainly the case of Michael Jackson (1958–2009) argues for a popular understanding of the face as the mirror of the soul. Michael Jackson had multiple surgeries. One of the sets of photographs that circulated after his death documents his startling transformation over time. His nose seems to grow ever thinner, his skin ever lighter.

The images have spawned thousands of diagnoses from armchair psychologists, most of them concluding that he was self-hating, uncomfortable with his ethnicity or his gender or both. Central to this notion was a sense of the inauthenticity of his appearance. *Los Angeles Times* columnist Tim Rutten observed that Jackson "was best known for his bizarre life, obsession with cosmetic surgery and for the allegations of pedophilia against him."[34] Even his advocates called this a sign of his mental instability: "We treated him like a carnival freak. We viewed his nose and his skin color as entertainment, not evidence of extreme mental illness."[35] Jackson's soul is seen to be mirrored in his desire to change his outward appearance. As both the surgeons and the psychoanalysts of the late nineteenth century were quick to point out, a desire to change one's appearance may result in the removal of a source of unhappiness. However, they would also contest that a desire to change one's appearance is neither evidence of psychopathology or, indeed, a guarantee of happy authenticity.

Historically, patients seeking repeated aesthetic surgery was seen as evidence of possible psychopathology. In the late nineteenth century, the first modern cosmetic surgeons such as the American surgeon Robert F. Weir (1838–1894) were horrified when patients on whom they had operated came back for further procedures. In his 1892 paper on "sunken noses," Robert F. Weir (1838–1894) presented a case of "monomania" focusing on the nose.[36] The nose that Weir repaired was a nose that was "unduly large." The male patient came to Weir in 1887 "perturbed in mind concerning the unsightliness of his nose." This was not merely a "cosmetic annoyance," but "his physicians and relatives [saw it as] essential to the preservation of the balance of his mind." The shape of the nose was altered by the removal of a section of the septum intranasally. Weir reports that "The patient's mental relief was correspondingly great for a time." A few months after the correction, the patient returned wanting the nose to be reshaped. This was done with an incision, which altered the form of the base of the nose. A year later the patient returned for another operation. Weir initially refused "because I considered it a first-class nose as it was" but was again persuaded by his patient's family.[37] A further intranasal operation followed. Weir was perplexed that the surgeon's intervention, which created a "normal" nose, was not sufficient for the patient.

In the 1930s, the urge for multiple surgeries was given a label —"poly-surgical addiction"—by one of the leading American psychoanalysts, Karl A. Menninger (1893–1990). The term was used to describe those patients, including aesthetic surgical patients, who seemed to have a compulsive need for surgical interventions.[38] Menninger's view that the desire for multiple surgeries can constitute an "addiction" was echoed by many surgeons, such as the leading British cosmetic surgeon of World War I, Harold Delf Gillies, who, as we have seen, agreed with the psychological model. And indeed today the odd and often misused category of contemporary American psychiatry's *DSM-5* (2013), "Body Dysmorphic Disorder," suggests that repeated surgeries are evidence of some underlying psychopathology as it is defined as focusing on

> one or more perceived defects or flaws in physical appearance that are not observable or appear only slight to others, and by repetitive behaviors (e.g., mirror checking, excessive grooming, skin picking, or reassurance seeking) or mental acts (e.g., comparing one's appearance with that of other people) in response to the appearance concerns.[39]

Such patients flock to cosmetic surgeons in order to "rectify their imagined or slight defect" and may "eventually possess 'synthetic' noses, ears, breasts, hips, or other body parts."[40] It is listed as a somatization disorder that claims that underlying such an obsession with the body must be a psychopathology that causes

> impaired psychosocial functioning because of their appearance concerns. Impairment can range from moderate (e.g., avoidance of some social situations) to extreme and incapacitating (e.g., being completely housebound). On average, psychosocial functioning and quality of life are markedly poor.[41]

But of course one person's "slight defect" is another's massive problem; one person's "synthetic" nose is another's answer to unhappiness.[42] Today's intervention of choice is not surgery but rather anti-depressants.

Regarding the case of Michael Jackson, there is some evidence, according to Arnold Klein, Jackson's dermatologist, that Jackson suffered from a patchy bleaching of the skin called vitiligo. Vitiligo occurs in all races but is most evident in those with the darkest complexions.[43] If Jackson did suffer from this condition, he may have undergone skin-lightening procedures in an attempt to minimize the splotchiness. Yet even this attempt at reconstructive rather than cosmetic surgery was read as a sign of inauthenticity by African American commentators:

> By the time Jackson died, he was perhaps whiter than any white man that you know. Those who looked at the constant stream of replayed televised interviews, at the pale skin, the thin lips painted red, the straight hair, saw in his face the psychological wound that has scarred so many in the black community.
>
> You line up his album covers, from "Got to Be There" when he was 13 and brown with a big-tooth grin, to "Off the Wall," when he still had a beautiful nose and a big Afro, to "Thriller," when his skin was still beautiful brown, but his nose was smaller, to "Bad," when his nose was even thinner and his skin was white. You trace your finger over the transformation, looking for a clue as to why the lips changed, the nose became more upturned, the brown skin faded until it was bleached beyond recognition. . . .
>
> Jackson has insisted that his skin faded as the result of vitiligo, a condition that damages the skin's pigment. But experts say that condition leaves the skin spotted and blotchy. To the outer world, Jackson's skin appeared consistently white. And before-and-after photos of Jackson tell a deeper story about color discrimination, also known as colorism—an intra-racial discrimination among African Americans.[44]

Here and elsewhere Jackson's surgical reshaping of his nose is attributed, at least in part, to a racially based self-loathing. But that's not necessarily what it was. One of the things that the earliest cosmetic surgeons understood was that psychological discomfort with specific aspects of one's appearance is not necessarily a psychiatric disorder. Even before Hitler gained power, some Jews in Germany certainly changed their appearance to allow them to pass in societies that wrongly saw the shape of their ears or noses as indicators of their inferiority, as did some Irish in America during the nineteenth and twentieth centuries. In the Reconstruction era, African Americans had operations for the correction of so-called "parrot noses," and these procedures continue today. Certainly many of those were undertaken by light-skinned individuals wishing to pass as white, but should a desire to escape repression really be viewed as a pathology? Social marginalization can indeed cause unhappiness. The amelioration of this unhappiness is not necessarily a sign of the striving for a pathological happiness.

Most people today opt for surgery or other cosmetic treatments out of a simple desire to look their best—not to guarantee their happiness. Today Vietnamese Americans undertake nose jobs and double eyelid surgery not to "pass" but to change specific aspects of their appearance for the sake of standards of beauty that are as much "Asian" as they are "American." American Jews have nose jobs not to look "less Jewish" but to more closely approximate the beauty norms of the society in which they live. Indeed, there seems to be little correlation between ethnic identity and surgery in today's America. Some American Jews have surgery and see themselves as Jewish in the public sphere. Ethnic-specific plastic surgery is now commonplace—and it is usually not motivated by a desire to pass so much as a desire to improve one's self-image. Just look at the growing popularity of chemical facelifts such as Botox, which is now widely used by men as well as women. Most of those who get the treatments aren't self-hating, aren't trying to pass for twenty; they just want to look good for their age.[45] Is that inauthenticity or simply the amelioration of unhappiness?

Today we have evolved a wide range of aesthetic procedures that claim to produce a body that is psychologically healthy. Yet the debate remains as to whether they produce an authentic face and a healthier psyche or are decried as unnecessary and the product of a false consciousness. Today, the anxiety about facial allotransplants as "inauthentic" reflects the anxiety about the fluidity of identity and its "rootedness" in the body. All present and potential changes to the face are questioned as "inauthentic" until they become the new "authentic." Why are we what we are? As Karen Barad observes, "We are responsible for the world of which we are a part, not because it is an arbitrary construction of our choosing but because reality is sedimented out of particular practices that we have a role in shaping and through which we are shaped."[46] The face is one of the sites for that shaping, literally and figuratively.

Notes

1. See my two studies *Creating Beauty to Cure the Soul: Race and Psychology in the Shaping of Aesthetic Surgery* (Durham: Duke University Press, 1998); *Making the Body Beautiful: A Cultural History of Aesthetic Surgery* (Princeton: Princeton University Press, 1999).

2. Michael H. Kernis and Brian M. Goldman, "A Multicomponent Conceptualization of Authenticity: Theory and Research," *Advances in Experimental Social Psychology* 38 (2006): 283–357, here 283.
3. Art Carey, "Men's faces go under the knife," *The Philadelphia Inquirer* (February 19, 2006), M02.
4. One can certainly add breast augmentation to this list when it becomes popular after WWII. But the fact that breast reconstruction is not so labeled even though the procedures are for the most part identical to breast augmentation, places this in a unique place to judge the meaning of "authenticity" in aesthetic surgery.
5. Stephan Mencke, *Zur Geschichte der Orthopädie* (Munich: Michael Beckstein, 1930), 68–69.
6. Hans F. K. Günther, *Rassenkunde des jüdischen Volkes* (München: J. F. Lehmann, 1930), 218.
7. Telemachus Thomas Timayenis, *The Original Mr. Jacobs* (New York: The Minerva Publishing Co., 1888), 21. See Michael Selzer, ed., *"Kike!": A Documentary History of Anti-Semitism in America* (New York: World Publishing, 1972), plate 16.
8. Jack E. Davis and Horacio H. Hernandez, "History of the Aesthetic Surgery of the Ear," in Mario González-Ulloa, ed., *The Creation of Aesthetic Plastic Surgery* (New York: Springer, 1976), 115–35.
9. "Über die operative Verkleinerung einer Nase (Rhinomiosis)," *Berliner klinische Wochenschrift* 40 (1898): 882–85. Translation from Jacques Joseph, "Operative Reduction of the Size of a Nose (Rhinomiosis)," trans. Gustave Aufricht, *Plastic and Reconstructive Surgery* 46 (1970): 178–81, here 178.
10. Joseph, "Operative Reduction," 180.
11. Jacques Joseph, *Nasenplastik und sonstige Gesichtsplastik, nebst einem Anhang über Mammaplastik und einige weitere Operationen aus dem Gebiete der äusseren Körperplastik: Ein Atlas und ein Lehrbuch* (Leipzig: C. Kabitzsch, 1931). All quotations are from the translation by Stanley Milstein, Jacques Joseph, *Rhinoplasty and Facial Plastic Surgery with a Supplement on Mammaplasty and Other Operations in the Field of Plastic Surgery of the Body* (Phoenix: Columella Press, 1987), here 34.
12. Ibid., 35.
13. Cited by Blair Rogers, "John Orlando Roe—Not Jacques Joseph—the Father of Aesthetic Rhinoplasty," *Aesthetic Plastic Surgery* 10 (1986): 63–88, here 81.
14. Jacques Joseph, "Nasenverkleinerung (mit Krankenvorstellung)," *Deutsche Medizinische Wochenschrift* 30 (1904): 1095. See also his "Nasenverkleinerungen," *Verhandlungen der deutsche Gesellschaft für Chirugie* 33 (1904): 112–20 as well as *Eine Nasenplastik, ausgeführt* in *Lokalanesthesie* (Berlin: G. Stilke, 1927).
15. Theodor Herzl, "Neue Nasen" in *Die treibende Kraft: Feuilltons*, ed., Markus G. Patka (Vienna: Picus, 2004), pp. 54–61. See also Peter Hyöng, "A Dream of a White Vienna after World War I: Hugo Bettauers *The City Without Jews* and *The Blue Stain*," in La Vinia Delois Jennings, ed., *At Home and Abroad: Historicizing Twentieth-Century Whiteness in Literature and Performance* (Knoxville: University of Tennessee Press, 2009), 29–60.

16. A review of the 28 face transplants to date has been undertaken at New York University Langone Medical Center. See Saami Khalifian, Eduardo D. Rodriguez, et al., "Facial Transplantation: The First 9 Years," *The Lancet* (on line 27 April 2014).
17. Craig S. Smith, "As a Face Transplant Heals, Flurries of Questions Arise," *The New York Times*, December 14, 2005, A1.
18. The technical nature of transplantation is not in question here; rather the cultural bias that sees the nature of transplantation not as a technical but rather as an ethical question. Concerning the first see Thomas Schlich, *The Origins of Organ Transplantation: Surgery and Laboratory Science, 1880–1930* (Rochester, NY: University of Rochester Press, 2010) and François Delaporte, Emmanuel Fournier, and Bernard Devauchelle, *La Fabrique du visage. De la physiognomonie antique à la première greffe. Avec un inédit de Duchenne de Boulogne* (Paris, Editions Brepols, coll. De Diversis Artibus, 2010).
19. Raffi Khatchadourian, "Transfiguration: How Dallas Wiens found a New Face," *The New Yorker* 88, no. 1, February 13, 2012, 70.
20. This is not unique to the Amien group. See Maria Z. Siemionow, *Face To Face: My Quest To Perform The World's First Full Face Transplant* (New York: Kaplan, 2009).
21. Khatchadourian, "Transfiguration."
22. I am indebted to the work of Carla Bluhm; Nathan Clendenin, *Someone Else's Face In The Mirror: Identity And The New Science Of Face Transplants* (Westport, Connecticut: Praeger, 2009).
23. Tim Radford, "Scientists ready for first full-face transplant," *Manchester Guardian Weekly*, June 4, 2004 - June 10, 2004, 170, no. 24, 7. On the question of the ethics of face transplants see C. A. T. Durrant, "Principilism And The Ethics Of Facial Transplantation (master's thesis, University of Wales, Lampeter, 2010) and Robert Lane, "Evaluation Of The Ethics Involved In Facial Transplantation," (master's thesis, KCUMB, 2010).
24. Anon., "Behind the Mask: Face transplant Reveals Mystery of Identity," *The Dallas Morning News* [Texas], December 8, 2005, editorial page.
25. Stephen Kiehl, "Her New Face Gives Woman a 'Normal Life,'" *The Baltimore Sun*, February 7, 2006,1C.
26. Ayesha Nathoo, *Hearts Exposed: Transplants and the Media in 1960s Britain* (Basingstoke: Palgrave Macmillan, 2009).
27. Dr. Danny Penman, "Can we really transplant a human soul?" *Daily Mail* (London), April 9, 2008, 14.
28. The answer here is simply no: Gesine Göschel, *Die Geschichte der Hornhauttransplantation* (Marburg an der Lahn: Basilisken-Presse, 1992).
29. See also Susan Whitman Helfgot; William Novak, *The Match: Complete Strangers, A Miracle Face Transplant, Two Lives Transformed* (New York: Simon & Schuster, 2010).
30. Judy Montagu, "A Question of Identity," *Jerusalem Post*, April 11, 2012, 14.
31. P. Pirnay, C. Herve, J.-P. Meningaud, "Des premières réimplantations aux premières transplantations totales de la face : l'histoire de prouesses chirurgicales," *Revue De Stomatologie Et De Chirurgie Maxillo-faciale* 112, no. 2 (2011): 93–100.

32. Robert Hanks, "The Hardest Graft Of All," *The Independent* (London), June 25, 2004, 33.
33. Tania Ewing, "The team that saved the face that sewed the arm," *The Age* (Melbourne, Australia), October 11, 1997, 4.
34. Tim Rutten, "Culture of celebrity has crossed over into political arena," *Los Angeles Times*, Sunday, July 12, 2009, E2.
35. Christine Stapleton, "Jackson's Death Should Raise Awareness of Illness," *Palm Beach Post* (Florida), Sunday July 5, 2009, 3D.
36. Robert F. Weir, "On Restoring Sunken Noses without Scarring the Face," *New York Medical Journal* 56 (1892): 449–454.
37. Ibid., 141–2.
38. Karl A. Menninger, "Polysurgery and Polysurgical Addiction," *Psychoanalytic Quarterly* 3 (1934): 173–199.
39. American Psychiatric Association, *Diagnostic and Statistical Manual of Mental Disorders, Fifth* Edition (Washington, D.C.: American Psychiatric Publishing, 2013), here 236.
40. DSM-IV, 509.
41. DSM-5, 245.
42. The *Diagnostic and Statistical Manual[s] of Mental Disorders* of the American Psychiatric Association are the standard American (and in general now global) diagnostic criteria for mental illness. In addition to the fifth edition in 2013, it has appeared in five different editions. *Diagnostic and Statistical Manual of Mental Disorders* (Washington, D.C.: American Psychiatric Association, 1st ed., 1952]; 2nd. ed. [1968]; 3rd ed. [1980]; 3rd ed.-R[evised] [1987]; 4th ed. [1994]; text revised 4th ed. [2000]). Here all of the quotations are from DSM-5, pp. 507–10; section 300.7. On DSM-III and aesthetic surgery see Louis Linn, "Cosmetic Surgery, with Particular Reference to Rhinoplasty," in Richard S. Blacher, ed., *The Psychological Experience of Surgery* (New York: John Wiley & Sons, 1987), 194–206.
43. "Jackson, healthy or not? Depends on who's talking," *The Associated Press*, July 13, 2009.
44. DeNeen L. Brown, "Through the Past, Darkly; The Legacy of Colorism Reflects Wounds of Racism That Are More Than Skin-Deep," *The Washington Post*, Sunday, July 12, 2009, E01.
45. See my "Aesthetic Anthropology," *Aesthetic Buyers Guide* (November 2007): 81–89.
46. Karen Barad, *Meeting the Universe Halfway* (Durham, NC: Duke University Press, 2006), 390.

Questions

Why are our faces so important in defining who we are?

What does authenticity mean?

Is altering the body a violation or an affirmation of "human rights"?

What are the guidelines for a successful face transplant?

Does altering your face mean you are altering your character?

Case Three

Posture and Health

Problems: Our bodies are malleable. They change with age and with the demands that we place on them. Our bodies may well be inherently different at birth from our bodies at the end of life. How we stand—our posture—defines us as healthy or ill, able or disabled, beautiful or ugly. It defines us as human or not human. How do these shifting ideas of posture provide insights into the claims society makes on who we are and what we are able to do?

This case study presents a set of interlinked claims about posture in modern culture. Over the past two centuries, posture has come to define a wide range of assumptions in the West from what makes human beings human (from Lamarck to Darwin and beyond) to the efficacy of the body in warfare (from Dutch drill manuals in the seventeenth century to German military medical studies of soldiers in the nineteenth century). Dance and sport both are forms of posture training in terms of their own claims. Posture separates 'primitive' from 'advanced' peoples and the 'ill' from the 'healthy.' Indeed an entire medical sub-specialty developed during the nineteenth century in which gymnastics defined and recuperated the body. But all of these claims were also part of a Western attempt to use posture (and the means of altering it) as the litmus test for the healthy modern body of the perfect citizen. Focusing on the centrality of posture in two oddly linked moments of modern thought—modern Zionist thought and Nationalism in early-twentieth-century China—in terms of bodily reform, we see how "posture" brings together the earlier debates to reform the body.

Entangled Genealogies

Certainly even the remembered whisper of "stand up straight" brings us to attention. Whether uttered by parent, teacher, or sergeant, it is a call to be self-aware or at least aware of how we are seen. Posture, that code for the way that we stand, is used over and over again as marker for a way to be. Over the past two centuries, it has come to define a

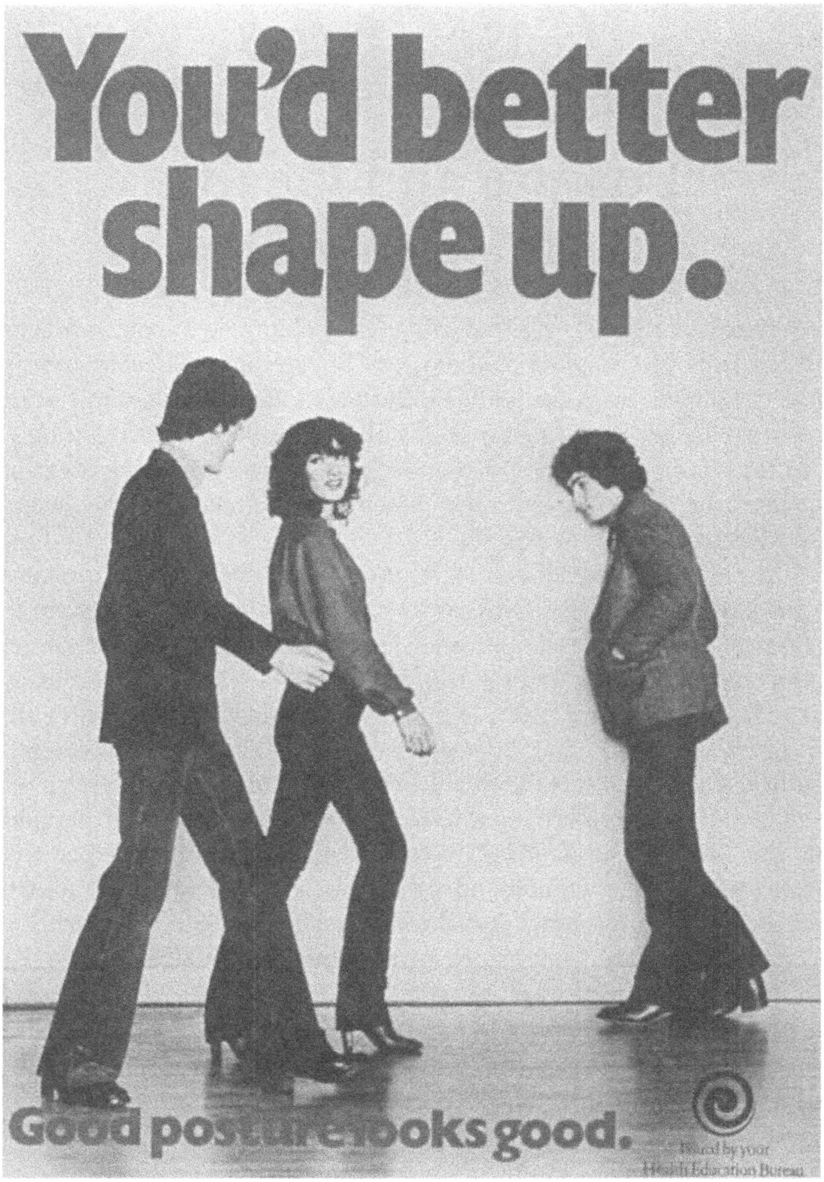

Figure 3.1. Public health authorities interested themselves in good posture as a sign of good psychological health in the 1960s. Image credit: National Library of Medicine Poster Collection.

wide range of truths: from what makes human beings human to the efficacy of the body in warfare and sport to ideas of health and illness in nineteenth-century biology and medicine.[1] We are the way we stand—ideally. Yet posture is not a fixed concept: it is understood as either part of fixed physiognomy, the inherent structures of the body, determined by inheritance, or of mobile physiognomy, determined by either pathology or by culture. We stand the way we do because of either "nature" or "nurture" in these views, and they define the universe of concepts into which we as human beings are to be comprehended. We are, as Karen Barad notes, "responsible for the world of which we are a part, not because it is an arbitrary construction of our choosing but because reality is sedimented out of particular practices that we have a role in shaping and through which we are shaped."[2] Posture is defined by the "entangled genealogies"[3] of the various uses and meanings associated with the very term "posture" and not necessarily by the claims of those who define what posture is to be.

Posture is a fluid concept that moves regularly between "statics" (the position of the body in rest), "mechanics" or "gait" (how the body moves in space and time), and those activities such as "sport," "dance," or "drill" (the cultural organization of both static and mechanic movement). Posture represents inherently entangled discourses. While we can begin with statics, this concept of posture is impacted by the rules by which one should sit, stand, and present oneself in social situations in order to become "human" and then a "modern," civilized citizen. Take the Anglophone understanding of posture, for instance. The OED defines posture in multiple ways that are inherently entangled. The root of the word is the French posture—meaning the position of the body—that is documented from 1588 in Middle French and then in 1580 as *posteure* in a figurative use, which in turn has its origin in classical Latin *positura*. As in French, its first meaning is as:

> the relative disposition of the various parts of something; *esp.* the position and carriage of the limbs or the body as a whole, often as indicating a particular quality, feeling, etc.; an attitude, a pose. Hence, more generally: the manner in which a person bears himself or herself; natural carriage or deportment.

It is the phrase "natural carriage or deportment" that captures the core problem of the term. The way one "naturally" appears is the way one acts. Sir Philip Sidney's *The Countesse of Pembrokes Arcadia* (1586) is listed by the OED as the first usage: "In another table was Atalanta; the posture of whose lims was so liuelie expressed, that if the eyes were the only iudges, . . . one would haue sworne the very picture had runne." A generation later in 1616, William Shakespeare in *Anthony and Cleopatra* uses it quite freely: "I shall see Some squeaking Cleopatra

Boy my greatnesse I' th' posture of a Whore." What is striking is that the military meaning of posture as "a particular position of a weapon, or a method of wielding it, in drill or battle" is documented as early as 1611 in W. Strachey's *For Colony of Virginea Britannia. Lawes Diuine, Morall & Martiall:* "Concerning the training, and cleanely exercising of their Armes, & their postures, the captains shall haue order and directions for the same vnder the Marshals hand." Very quickly even the figurative meaning as "a mental or spiritual attitude or condition" takes on its military implications in 1642 in the very title of J. Taylor's *An Apology for Private Preaching whereunto is annexed the Spirituall postures, alluding to that of Musket and Pike.* Indeed, it is striking that thereafter the military meaning colors all future usage. The political meaning of posture as "a state of being; a condition or situation in relation to circumstances" is also present in English from the seventeenth century, as in a 1620 letter from Sir Henry Wotton: "We stood thus in a posture of affairs . . . very favourable." The scientific meaning of posture as it is used in contemporary scientific papers is a twentieth-century use, but there is an obsolete scientific meaning as "the position of a thing (or person) relative to another; position, situation" documented as early as 1605 in Francis Bacon's *The twoo bookes of Francis Bacon: Of the proficience and aduancement of learning, diuine and humane*: "In describing the fourmes of Vertue and Duty, with their situations and postures, in distributing them into their kinds, parts, Prouinces."[4] Posture thus has multiple, overarching meanings that exemplify the entangled genealogies inherent in any understanding of the human body.

The idealized upright static and mechanical posture in the early modern West seems to have originated in the late sixteenth-century with both the development and representation of military drill formation. The break at this historical point in the meaning of drilling soldiers seems obvious to military historians.[5] Its impact on the use of the term was immediate. Posture is thus at its origin a quality and an image ascribed to men. Jacob de Gheyn's 117 illustrations for *The Exercise of Armes* (1607) present images of close order drill from Maurice of Orange's drill manual of the late 1590s, *Wapen-handelinghe van roers, musquetten, en spiessen,* that show the optimum positions for carrying and shooting or using weapons (Parker 2007). The resting position or "attention" is the basis for the "ideal" posture. This ideal or rest position is what comes to be "standing at attention" with a more or less rigid spine, tucked-in chin, and feet clearly positioned under the head, back but yet not rigidly aligned with the rest of the body. The "plumb line" from the top of the head to the feet is present. All of the other positions illustrated by de Gheyn are functional—they instruct the reader/viewer on how to hold the musket (or pike) in a series of positions that enables units of soldiers to volley fire or charge.[6]

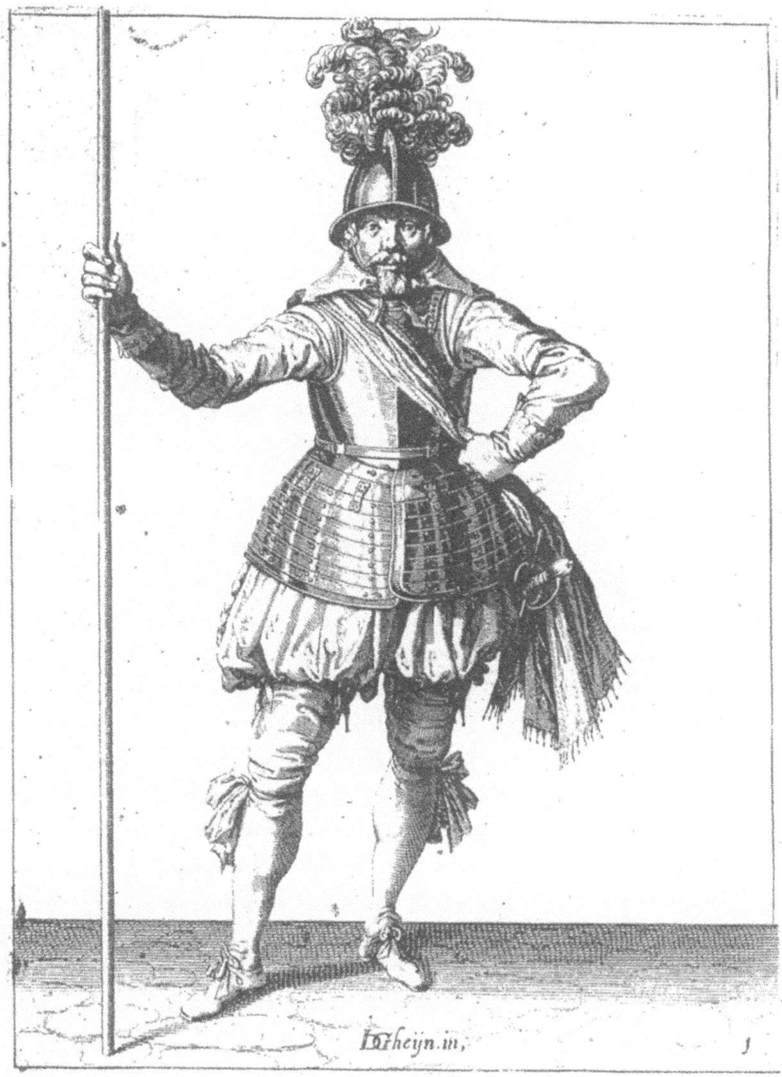

Figure 3.2. The pike man at rest from Jacob de Gheyn's *Wapenhandelinghe Van Roers: Mvsqvetten Ende Spiessen. Achtervolgende De Ordre Van Sÿn Excellentie Maurits, Prince Van Orangie, Graue Van Nassau, Etc., Gouverneur Ende Capiteÿn Generael Ouer Gelderlant, Hollant, Zeelant, Vtrecht, Overÿssel, Etc.* (The Hague: Gedruckt int SGrauen, 1607).

The Nassau drill manual was intended to show how to load, shoot, and reload in unison, and therefore each movement had to be precise and was frozen in time in de Gheyn's 117 illustrations (Roodenburg 1997). But the sense is that the body of the soldier must mirror the rigidity of the weapon. Indeed the very term for such drill books is a "posture book," as in 1631 when Ben Jonson in his drama *The divell is an asse* observes that they must:

> And by the vertue' of those, draw downe a wife
> There from a windo', worth ten thousand pound!
> Get him the posture booke, and's leaden men,
> To set vpon a table, 'gainst his Mistresse
> Chance to come by, that hee may draw her in,
> And shew her *Finsbury* battells.[7]

By 1691 such use comes to be commonplace: "He learned . . . how to handle the pike and musquet, and all postures belonging to them."[8] Posture is clearly defined; posture is visually represented; posture is manly, erect, and upright.

Over the next century, the rest position itself is so altered that by 1791 it is more rigidly aligned, with the feet together rather than apart and the spine rigidly erect.[9] The plumb line itself evolved over time. This was clearly never a natural position; it was learned and rehearsed until all soldiers at attention looked identical. This position came to define the military body and through the meanings attached to it, the normal, healthy individual. The military positions are analogous to the dance positions of the eighteenth century: clearly unnatural and having a specific function only within the movements required for the exercise. Posture in dance and the military seem to be interrelated, not, as William H. McNeill, claimed because such organized movement reflects the intuitive imperative of the beating heart translated into action, but because of normative positions of what is acceptable defined here as functional posture in any given setting. While McNeill is interested in movement to music, his own project has yet another source. He writes of his experience of "swaggering in conformity with prescribed military postures" and of this leading to a "strange sense of personal enlargement; a sort of swelling out, becoming bigger than life, thanks to participation in collective ritual."[10] Drill and drill position have meaning; the military posture comes to define a collectivity in very specific ways.

Michel Foucault contrasts the premodern soldier with that of the modern age. In *Discipline and Punish* he characterizes the former as: "... someone who could be recognized from afar; he bore certain signs: the natural signs of his strength and his courage, the marks, too, of his pride; his body was the blazon of his strength and valour."[11] Such a soldier has a body that reflects the untaught and natural (according to his view): "an erect head, a taut stomach, broad shoulders, long arms, strong fingers, a small belly, thick thighs, slender legs and dry feet."[12] The modern solider, that of the soldier who is trained and shaped by the military manual is quite different: "By the late eighteenth century," he writes, "the soldier has become something that can be made; out of a formless clay, an inapt body, the machine required can be constructed; posture is gradually corrected; a calculated constraint runs slowly through each part of the body, mastering it, making it pliable."[13] The soldier whose body is defined by his posture "that maybe subjected, used, transformed and improved."[14]

But the person who trains the body moves in the course of the eighteen century from the military into civilian life. He is the "posture master." Samuel Johnson's dictionary defines him as "one who teaches or practices artificial contortions of the body," citing *The Spectator*.[15] The vogue for such training began with the visit to London by Tiberio Fiorillo, a Neapolitan actor known for his interpretation of Scaramouche, at the end of the seventeenth century. But the idea remains within British society through at least Sir Walter Scott's novel *Kenilworth* (1821), "where a gentleman may break his neck if he does not walk as upright as a posture-master on the tight-rope."[16] Artificial and highly shaped bodies are no longer limited to the drill ground but are found now in better society, if only as the object of amusement. Here the erect body becomes a standard by which a rising middle class (in the army and in the drawing room) can perform as if their bodies were no longer marked as different from the elites.

By 1889, the Leipzig anatomist Christian Wilhelm Braune and his student Otto Fischer dropped the plumb line along the now acceptable rigid posture of "standing at attention," bringing the study of military posture into the medical literature.[17] Their statistical measurements of body posture remain the basis for all contemporary discussions of the "straight line inside the body" within the various sciences of posture from orthopedics to military medicine.[18] Rooted in Braune's complex analysis of the center of gravity in human anatomy, the study of posture is an attempt to translate such knowledge into a mechanical

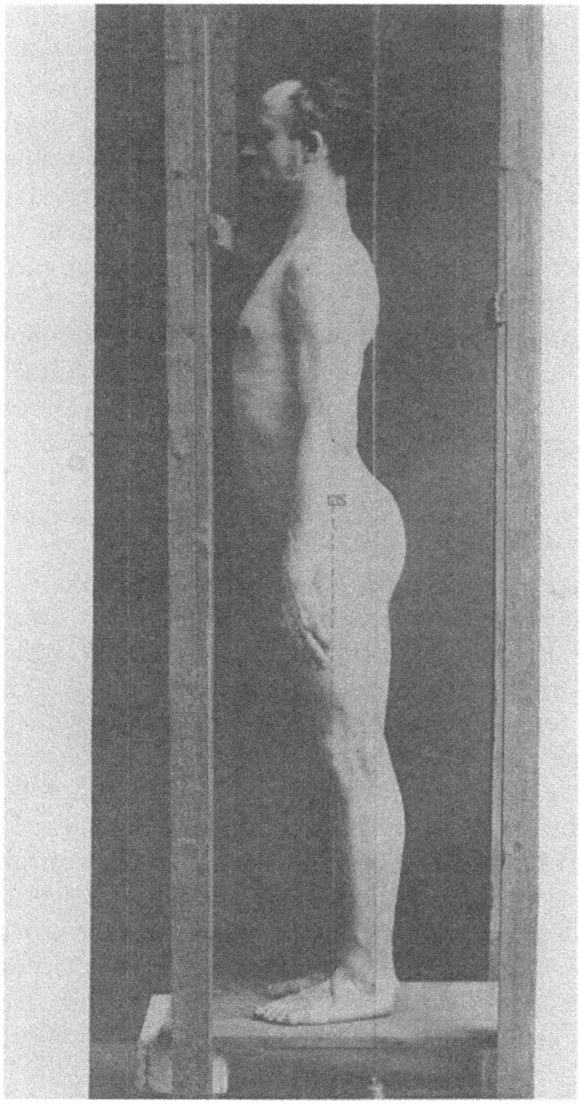

Figure 3.3. The plumb line with a plumb bob from Christian Wilhelm Braune and Otto Fischer, *Über den Schwerpunkt des menschlichen Körpers mit Rücksicht auf die Ausrüstung des deutschen Infanteristen* (Leipzig: S. Hirzel, 1889).

profile of what the upright body can be made to do under optimum circumstances and to define those circumstances. They quite easily use the concept of the plumb line, employing an actual plumb bob as a given means of imagining the forces moving throughout the body.

For them the body is always dynamic but must be understood as having a maximum productive stance for specific undertakings.[19] The science of posture results from this moment in military medicine. "Stand up straight" may not have first arisen in the military (parents might well have that priority), but its first codified and visual documentation is in this world, and the military origin of upright posture informs later discussions of posture as a quality not of men but of human beings.

Certainly the idea of upright posture and upright character haunted the Prussian court, setting the tone for Braune and Fischer's work. Kaiser Wilhelm II hired the American body culturist Elizabeth Marguerite de Varel Mensendieck (c. 1866–1959), better known as Bess M. Mensendieck, to improve the posture of his courtiers:

> The potbellies of the ladies-in-waiting of the last German imperial court always annoyed Kaiser Wilhelm II. In an effort to appease him, whenever they stood at attention in his presence they folded their hands over their bulging abdomens. This posture made them look like fantastic beer-mugs, a sight which vexed Wilhelm further. Hearing that a sturdy little blonde U. S. esthete named Bess M. Mensendieck taught men & women how to stand and move gracefully, by means of what she called "functional exercises," he summoned her to do the same for his court. Cried the Kaiser: "They are the most awkward women in the world. One never sees women at the courts of London, St. Petersburg or Rome stand about in the graceless attitudes I see at mine."[20]

Her correct posture is one we have seen before:

> When the human animal stands properly erect, an imaginary line should cut the nose, chin, breastbone and crotch. Another imaginary line should drop from the mastoid, in front of the shoulder joint, through the elbow and little finger (palm turned to the rear), side of knee and ankle. This is achieved by standing with feet together, shoulders held back, abdomen tucked in, buttocks clenched.[21]

Posture at the Origin of Human Beings

"Good" or "natural" posture and the plumb line separates "primitive" from "advanced" peoples as well as the "ill" from the "healthy" and even the "human" from "prehuman." When I was at university in the early 1960s, there were a number of characteristics taught that defined the uniqueness of human beings: language, the opposable thumb and the use of tools, consciousness, morality, emotions, and, last but not least, upright posture. Over the past decades, more and more of these qualities (correctly or not) have been shown as shared with any number of animals, from the primates to the anteater. Only upright posture has been maintained as the quality that defines the human, indeed, it has come has come to be the defining attribute that draws the evolutionary line between the earliest human beings and their predecessors. As a recent review of gait and posture states:

> Bipedality is commonly performed by a variety of primates and other mammals, even some artiodactyls. Human ancestors, however, adopted this odd gait as their exclusive form of locomotion, and so extensively modified their postcranium that every transport event, whether a simple stroll of a few yards or a desperate flight to avoid an attacking predator, became restricted to its use."[22]

We are our posture.

Recently the discovery of *Ardipithecus ramidus* has our ancient ancestor defined as an ancestor because of "upright walking":

> This remarkably rare skeleton is not the oldest putative hominin, but it is by far the most complete of the earliest specimens. It includes most of the skull and teeth, as well as the pelvis, hands, and feet—parts that the authors say reveal an 'intermediate' form of upright walking, considered a hallmark of hominins.[23]

The representation of this "ancestor" in the scholarly paper is of a hairy individual standing rigidly upright. Not only bipedalism, walking on two feet, and upright walking defines human ancestry but also standing up straight in an unspoken way. The reasons for this plumb line upright posture have recently been found in the unique geography of where these ancestors lived: it is now claimed that they stood upright because *Ardipithecus ramidus* "was a denizen of woodland with small patches of forest high grass."[24] One had to be able to look over the grass to see their prey—and standing straight seems to have been the way to do it. This claim answered Arthur Keith's view, which summarized Charles Darwin's perspective articulated in the 1920s that "it was on the trees, not on the ground, that man came by the initial stages of his posture and carriage."[25] To paraphrase Friedrich Nietzsche, *Ardipithecus ramidus's* posture was the result of what it ate or at least where it ate it.

In this view of upright posture, modern anthropology inherits the mantle of the ancient world. The very notion of what defines the human being in contrast to all other living things in the ancient world is simple: upright posture. As Marjorie O'Rourke Boyle has observed, the human being is defined across all aspects of classical thought as "standing on two feet support[ing] a straight spine."[26] Indeed, Aristotle says "man is the only being that stands upright"[27]:

> The human being is the only erect animal because its nature and essence is divine; the function of the most divine is thinking and being intelligent; and that is not easy when much of the body is pressing from above, for the weight makes thought and the common sense sluggish.[28]

Intelligence and upright posture is now linked for the first but not the last time, and upright posture is defined as bipedalism. How this is read differs from commentator to commentator. Best known of the ancient commentators is Plato, in the *Timaeus*, who sees man as bipedal and featherless, striving for the infinite and for knowledge.[29] *Anthropos*, the word for man, means the animal that looks upward and considers the gods. Although bipedalism seems comfortable to us, Plato moves the rational mind far away from the center of the appetite and from the organ of generation:

> As regards the most sovereign kind of soul in us, we must conceive of it in this way: god has given to each of us, as his daemon, that which we say resides in the summit of our body and which raises us from earth towards its kin in the heaven, since we are not an earthly but a heavenly plant, as they say most truly. For it is there, whence the soul first sprang into birth, that the divine [part of us] suspends our head or root and thus erects the whole body.[30]

The head for Plato is the "acropolis" of the body, its highest point both literally and metaphorically. Xenophon, in the *Memorabilia* (I.4.11), builds on the notion of the head as the body's acropolis takes a more functional view arguing that "In the first place, man is the only living creature that they have caused to stand upright; and the upright position gives him a wider range of vision in front and a better view of everything above and exposes him to less injury."[31] For the Greeks, the meaning associated with standing upright is part of a rhetoric of military defense, as the very idea of the acropolis is always understood as the space that is both defensible and which defines the new city-state as a national space. Man stands upright thus as metaphor for the human condition seeking the divine but also defending the human.

"Featherless" sounds odder to modern ears than does the functional association of bipedalism and intelligence, but Plato sees the absence of bodily covering as a move away from the base toward the human, for he is quite aware that the other bipedal animal is the bird. Greek thought attributes a middle role for the bird between man and the gods, as birds are connected with the gods through their use in divination. Responding to Plato's contorted definition, Diogenes the Cynic notoriously plucked a (bipedal) chicken and took it to Plato's Academy, declaring, "Here is Plato's man."[32] The followers of Plato responded by revising Plato's definition of a human being as a featherless biped, expanding it to include "with straight nails." For the ancient world, there was no question of the primacy of bipedal, upright man. As late at the Renaissance, Erasmus platonically continued to defined humans as "featherless and bipedal."

The claim that it is posture that defines a human being continues to the beginning of modernity when Johann Gottfried Herder in his *Ideas for the Philosophy of History of Humanity* (1784–1791) defines posture first and foremost as central to the "organic difference between man and beast." Yet, unlike the classical tradition, he discusses this before he discusses human reasoning.

> The form of man is upright: in this he is singular upon the earth. For though the bear has equally broad foot, and stands erect when he fights: though the ape and the pygmy sometimes walk or run in an erect posture: still to the human species alone is this position natural and constant. The foot of man is more form and broad: he has a great long toe, while the ape has but a thumb, his heel too is on a level with the sole of his foot. All the muscles acting in this position are adapted to it. The calf of the leg is enlarged: the pelvis is drawn backward: the hips are spread outwards from each other: the spine is less curved: the breast is widened: the shoulders have clavicles: the hands have fingers embued with the sense of feeling: to crown the structure the receding head is exalted on the muscles of the neck: man is . . . a creature looking far above and around him.[33]

This is the military posture, and the plumb line is now defined as human posture. Herder does not downplay the role of reason and above all speech, which one might expect, but the noble posture comes first with appropriate citations about the anatomical differences among animals to the anthropological literature of his time such as Thomas Camper and his son-in-law Theodor Soemmering as well as Johann Friedrich Blumenbach.[34] But Herder is, in the final analysis, a theologian. Upright posture is a sign of the very nature of creation crowned by an upright being whom God tells to "stand up straight":

> When our creative parent had fulfilled her labours, and exhausted all the forms, that were possible on our Earth, the paused, and surveyed her works: and as she saw, that the Earth still wanted it's [*sic*] principal ornament, it's [*sic*] regent, and second creator, she took counsel with herself, combined together her forms, and out of all fashioned her chief figure, human beauty. With maternal affection she stretched forth her hand to the last creature of her art, and said: "stand up on the earth! Left to thyself, thou hadst been a beast, like unto other beasts: but through my especial aid and love, *walk erect*, and be of beasts the god."
>
> With grateful eyes let us contemplate, in this hallowed act, the benefit, through which our race became a human species: with wonder shall we perceive, what new organism of powers commenced in the erect position of mankind, and how by it alone man was made a *man*. [35]

Herder's scientific sentiment bridges the gap between Plato's notion of upright posture signifying the seeking of the rational and John Milton's understanding that man's erect posture, created by the hand of God, preceded man's own intelligence:

> . . . a creature, who, not prone
> And brute as other creatures, but endued
> With sanctity of reason might erect
> His stature, and upright with front serene
> Govern the rest, self knowing; and from thence
> Magnanimous to correspond with Heaven,
> But grateful to acknowledge whence his good
> Descends, thither with heart, and voice, and eyes
> Directed in devotion to adore
> And worship God Supreme, who made him
> Of all his works . . . [36]

Human posture—for Herder standing upright and erect—is not only a divine gift but also a scientific attribute.

Immanuel Kant reacted against such a notion of the divine perfection of human posture and the theology that it implied. For him Herder's views are merely romantic psychologizing rather than an empirical statement of the nature of man and his future. Man is not perfect, but following very much from his understanding of what Enlightenment means, must have the potential to alter and change, "to use one's own mind without another's guidance. *Sapere aude.*"[37] For man "is himself an animal" as Kant observed in his *Idea for a Universal History with a*

Cosmopolitan Purpose (1784). There he characterized man as "crooked wood," from which "nothing perfectly straight can be built." Contemporary man is "stunted, crooked and twisted" and could attain a "beautiful, straight stature," but only as a goal after long years of effort, "for from such crooked wood as man is made of, nothing perfectly straight can be built."[38] Not divine perfection, not the reliance on pastors or physicians, but rigorous self-improvement creates good posture.

For Kant human self-improvement leads to the overcoming of our inherently crooked posture. One of his successors, in 1833, to the chair of philosophy at Königsberg, the Hegelian Rosenkranz, in his *Aesthetics of Ugliness* (*Aesthetik des Hässlichen*) (1853) argued precisely the opposite, that ugliness, the antithesis of beauty, resides in the totality of the essence of human existence on a scale that runs from the beautiful and intelligent to the "cretin who is yet even uglier than the Black, as they add to the unbalance of the body the stupidity of intelligence and the weakness of the spirit . . .":

> The ugly does not reside in the essence of human beings. Rather since rationality and freedom defines the human being, so too is it clear that being human is defined by the symmetry of the body, the differences in hands and feet, in human being's upright posture. Is a human being, like the Bushman or like the cretin, naturally ugly, such distortions of the body represent their local and relatively inherited lack of freedom. Disease is usually the source of ugliness when it distorts the skeleton, the bones and the muscles, as for example in syphilitic osteomyelitis or gangrenous destruction of the skeleton. It causes ugliness when it colors the skin, as in jaundice or covers the skin in ulcers as in scarlet fever, the plague and certain forms of syphilis. . . .[39]

Rosenkranz then easily moves from the aesthetic to the moral, seeing in ugliness the "origin of evil and the ugliness transmitted through evil to the external manifestation of human beings. Evil is not transcendent essence beyond the freedom of human beings."[40] It is the immutability of the body and its reflection of evil in its ugliness (whether in race, disability, or disease) that is defined by the lack of beautiful and therefore good posture.

The science of the post-Enlightenment agreed with Herder's sense that posture defined the human, without citing the act of creation, rather than agreeing with Kant's view of self-shaping. Jean-Baptiste Lamarck claimed at the opening of the nineteenth century that

> Indeed, if any race of primates (quadrumanes) whatsoever, particularly the more highly evolved of them, were to lose, either from force

> of circumstances or any other cause, the aptitude for tree climbing and of grasping the branches with their feet, as with their hands, for security of grip; and if the individuals of this race, for a series of generations, be obliged to use their feet only in walking, and cease using their hands as feet; then there is no doubt, from the evidence produced in the foregoing chapters, that these apes would finally be transformed into man (bimanes) and that the great toe, would no longer be separated from the other toes like a thumb, the feet serving merely the purposes of progression.[41]

For Lamarck, this posture is the result of human ancestors having left the trees for the open plain. But early evolutionary theory also sees human development in terms of race. Posture is one of the keys noted by nineteenth-century ethnologist Karl Hermann Burmeister in 1855, who commented that "Blacks and all of those with flat feet are closest to the animals."[42] Not too far from Herder's pygmies. Natural posture is primitive posture is bad posture; no plumb line.

Thomas Huxley picked this up in his image of the "natural" progression of the "Skeleton of the Gibbon, Orang, Chimpanzee, Gorilla

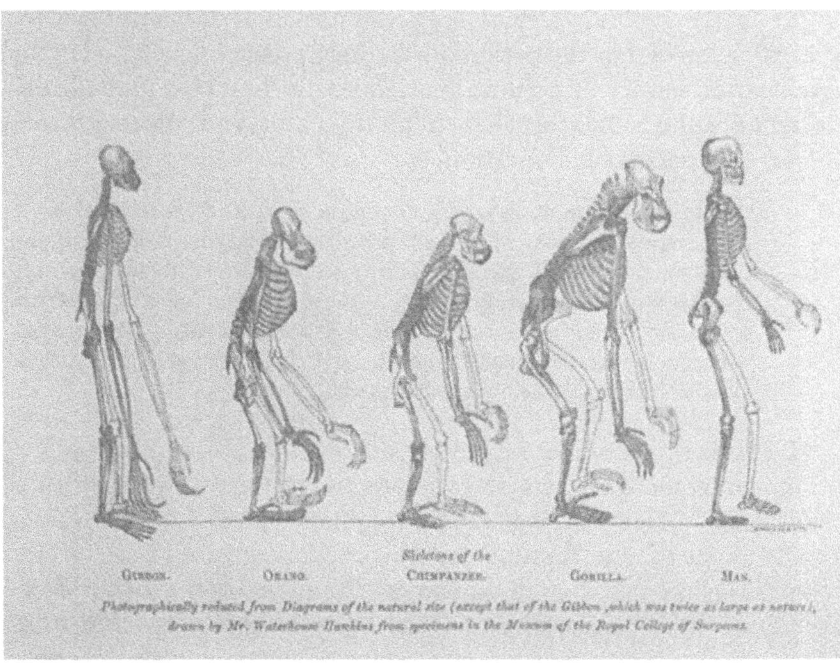

Figure 3.4. The often reproduced and even more often parodied progress of posture from gibbon to man from Thomas Huxley's 1863 *Evidence as to Man's Place in Nature* (London: Williams and Norgate, 1863).

and Man" in his 1863 *Man's Place in Nature*,[43] which meant that poor Neanderthal Man discovered in 1857 had (at least in the imagination of those who drew him) very poor posture—he was not quite human yet.[44] By the discovery of Pithecanthropus erectus's thighbone in 1891, there was no question that erect posture and assumed gait was the litmus test for evaluating the degree of "humanness" of the earliest ancestors. Why the evolution of erect posture? To no one's surprise, Charles Darwin's adaptation of Herbert Spencer's "survival of the fittest" in his *Descent of Man* (1871) meant that posture was determinant in survival:

> If it be an advantage to man to stand firmly on his feet and to have his hands and arms free, of which, from his pre-eminent success in the battle of life there can be no doubt, then I can see no reason why it should not have been advantageous to the progenitors of man to have become more and more erect or bipedal. They would thus have been better able to defend themselves with stones or clubs, to attack their prey, or otherwise to obtain food. The best built individuals would in the long run have succeeded best, and have survived in larger numbers.[45]

The "battle for life," Herbert Spencer's notion, is a replacement for and extension of the very notion of a military posture developed in the seventeenth century. The plumb line defines the "best built individuals." Upright posture is the most efficient for this battle, and correct posture defines the process of civilization. For

> . . . as the progenitors of man became more and more erect, with their hands and arms more and more modified for prehension and other purposes, with their feet and legs at the same time transformed for firm support and progression, endless other changes of structure would have become necessary. The pelvis would have to be broadened, the spine peculiarly curved, and the head fixed in an altered position, all which changes have been attained by man.[46]

All that is human is defined by the acquisition of upright posture.

One of the more engaged Darwinians and the creator of "historical materialism," Friedrich Engels, in a fragment of 1876 on the transition from ape to man through the need to work stressed that upright posture was the first step in human development, as it freed (following Darwin) the hands for work, and everything else resulted from this move to bipedalism. More radical than Darwin, Engels imagined that all aspects of human evolution begins with the development of bipedalism, while Darwin assumed that cognitive ability (and brain size) developed prior to bipedalism and led to it. Becoming human

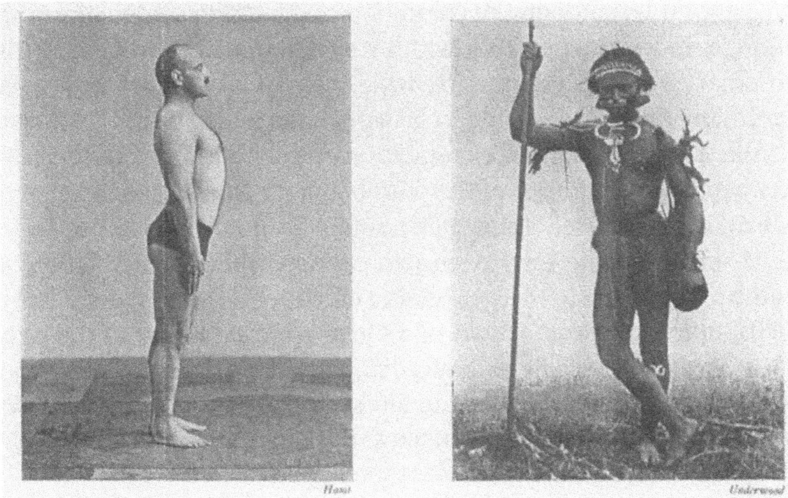

Figure 3.5. Civilized vs. natural posture. From F. A. Hornibrook, *The Cultures of the Abdomen* (London: Wm. Heinemann, 1927).

is the result of the specialization of the hands through work, "these apes began to lose the habit of using their hands to walk and adopted a more and more erect posture."[47] They began to "stand up straight"; indeed, Engels states, "this is the decisive step in becoming human."[48] This is the underlying rationale for the newest anthropological theories from Herder to the present defining the human being in terms of erect posture. Yet there are those who take a contrarian view. Upright posture has led to all of the cultural and physiological difficulties of modern human beings.

At mid-twentieth century, G. H. Estabrooks, a psychologist at Colgate, was clearly anti-Darwinian when it came to the course of human development. He was convinced that man began to deteriorate from the moment he adopted upright posture, arguing that the plague of bad sinuses in modern man is the result of his upright posture.[49] Becoming human means losing a connection to the "natural" body. This counter argument becomes a means of glorifying the "primitive" as being closer to the ideal or at least closer to nature. Science is, as Mitchell Ash argued, in a dynamic relationship with politics in which each serves as a resource for the other. Science may serve as a "cognitive, rhetorical or institutional resource" transforming its very content or practice in a political context.[50] In this manner, posture can serve as a litmus test for such transformation: anti-Darwinian views are also political positions.

Posture thus takes on the coloration of the political ideology of the moment. Indeed in the 1970s, with a very different notion of the history of human development, the left-wing theorist Klaus Theweleit questioned any positive meaning to be associated with upright (now read as military) posture in his examination of the notion of a relationship between fascist fantasies of the plumb line posture and masculinity.[51] In evoking "posture," Theweleit pointed to its extensive use in the racial science of the early twentieth century which denied "good" or plumb line posture to the weaker and corrupt "Eastern" races.[52] By the 1990s, upright posture is part of a philosophical fantasy of the right-wing German writer Peter Sloterdijk, who fantasizes the very act of awakening and sleepily swinging one's legs out of bed as our morning "ontogeny recapitulating phylogeny," of daily moving to bipedalism, upright posture, and transcendent intelligence:

> From the warm primal darkness primitive forms of the personality arise. Nobody has to tell me that the aim of the exercise is to achieve the vertical, even on this morning there is something in me ready to meet the generic fate that moved us to risk being on two legs and having free hands—head now available for considered perspective now placed at the highest point. No one can say is that I have not follow the call of human dignity this morning. The improbable—it now takes place, walking upright, it is the event, my standing there now on no more than two legs is an accomplished fact, is from now on it will be easy, easily to transverse the path of humanity to consciousness....[53]

Are we our posture, or are they *their* posture? This strikes me as the central question that reverberates down the history of posture.

Yet many scientists today continue to spin their notion of what makes man "man" around the development of upright posture and thus reveal the biases as to what actually defines the essential nature of the human being. Thus the controversy surrounding the American anthropologist C. Owen Lovejoy's claim in his 1981 monogamy-provisioning hypothesis, which imagined the earliest male evolved upright posture in order to be able to carry home food in his arms to his female mate while walking upright on his legs. All other evolutionary developments depart from this increase in efficiency. Lovejoy defines upright posture in a way that seems to be functional:

> Our upright posture, in contrast, places our center of mass almost directly over the foot. If we stand erect and lengthen our legs by straightening the knee and rotating the ankle, the ground reaction is directed vertically and we end up on tiptoe. In order to propel our

> upright trunk we must reposition our center of mass ahead of one leg. The trailing limb is lengthened to produce a ground reaction while the other leg is swung forward to keep the trunk from falling. The strength of the ground reaction is limited, because much of it is still directed vertically and also because the trailing limb is already near its limit of extension owing to our upright posture: the hip joint is fully extended and the knee joint nearly so.[54]

But the image of human posture contrasts the "PELVIS AND LEG of a chimpanzee (left) and a human being (right) reflect the differing demands of quadrupedal and bipedal locomotion."[55] It is as radical a representation as was Huxley's of the difference between prehuman and human, with the latter defined quite clearly by the plumb line representation of upright posture. This view of evolutionary efficiency caused an uproar in the first age of feminist thought, not because of its argument about the efficient male body, but because of its claim of the primacy of *male* evolution and monogamy.[56]

Posture, Disability, and Inheritance

In the nineteenth century, there was an entire medical subspecialty that defined the healthy body and treated the ill body based on notions of acceptable posture (think of this as a plumb line from Swedish gymnastics to German medical *Krankengymnastik* to modern gym culture). The range is almost always one that generates an image of the ideal posture, then moves to pathological postures such as the kyphotic and lordotic posture, flat-back posture, sway-back posture, and finally to the military posture as exaggeration of the ideal norm. Diagrams of the time show position of head (skull), neck (cervical vertebrae), thoracic and lumbar vertebrae, pelvis, leg (femur, tibia, fibula), and foot. Those are the anatomical features that define natural vs. pathological posture, just as there is the bright line between the prehuman and the human in terms of their upright posture. The categories of healthy vs. ill posture certainly have their roots in the medical understanding of correcting "poor" posture in cases of what was clearly defined as pathological posture such as the posture that results from vitamin deficiency diseases such as rickets (from vitamin D deficiency). Beginning with the first modern treatise of rickets—Daniel Whistler's 1684 *Disputatio medica inaugurales de morbo puerili Anglorum quem patrio idiômate indiginae vocant the rickets: quam Deo suppetias ferente*—there has been a focus on the posture of the sufferer. Thomas Levacher de la Feutrie, in his 1772 *Traité du rakitis, ou l'art de redresser les enfants contrefaits,* provides both exercises and implements to correct such pathologies.[57] The general sense is that rickets (called "the English malady") presents a manifest misshaping of the limbs in knock knees or bowed legs and in the earliest stages a so-called "tailorlike" posture, which is seen to mirror the position that a tailor takes in sewing. The very image of the child with rickets now having its body reformed, straightened, and corrected comes to define mechanical interventions in orthopedics, a medical discipline that uses instruments regularly to correct the body's malformation and, ideally, allow it to stand up straight. Disability in this sense is bad posture, and correction is demanded to return the disabled body to the plumb line. In doing so the claim is that the disabled body is made productive and returned to a meaningful role in a capitalist society in the form of an erect body.

Bad posture is not only a sign of physical pathology but also of moral degeneration. The form of the external body reflects character as well as psyche. By the time of Daniel Gottlob Moritz Schreber's *Die ärztliche Zimmergymnastik* (1855) the line between physical illness and moral position had become completely blurred (if it was ever clear). Schreber advocated both his "systematic remedial exercises" and countryside

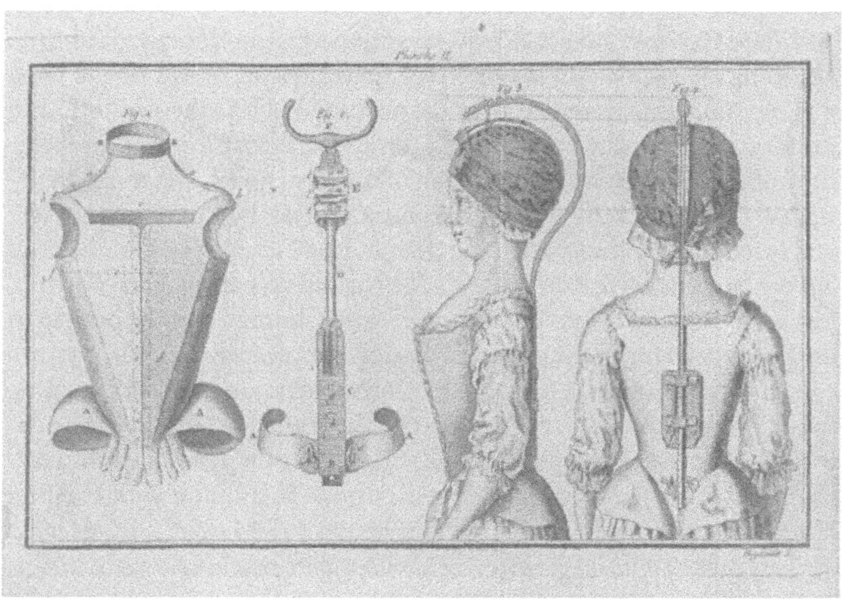

Figure 3.6 Correcting the posture of a patient with ricketts. Thomas Levacher de la Feutrie, *Traité du rakitis, ou l'art de redresser les enfants contrefaits* (Paris: Lacombe, 1772).

exercise for urban youth to overcome the problem of physical and moral degeneration. During his time, the term *Volksgesundheit* (people's health) was coined to reflect the inherent relationship between body and spirit. And in Germany, the very late appearance of the industrial revolution demanded that it would be a machine to correct bad posture. Thus it is not only exercise and training that corrects bad posture and bad minds, but also machines.

By the end of the century, 3.5 million copies of *Das neue Naturheilverfahren* (1888), by the German exponent of self-cure Friedrich Eduard Bilz, were sold to middle-class readers in Germany who were convinced that they had to learn to stand up straight. "Pathological" or "poor" was now clearly linked not only to the machines that corrected posture, but also to the machines that mimicked work. Think of the forerunners to our contemporary gym equipment that mimic bicycle riding or stair walking. Bilz's popular text advocated machines that mimicked factory or farm work. Good posture was accomplished by such imitated work; the good citizen's posture was the citizen who could contribute to the society by work or war.

Not only physical but also psychological states are revealed by posture. In Joseph Simms's 1887 *Physiognomy Illustrated,* he sets out a series of gaits and what they indicate about mental states. The "toddling gait," for example, indicated a helpless, childish man: "the toes of his shoes are much further out of repair than the heels; ... there are seldom all the buttons on the garments, and ... both a glove and an umbrella have just been lost; occasioning the necessity for trying to recollect every place Mr. Toddler has been."[58] He is contrasted with "Miss Mary Frisk." There was also a "plunging gait" where the walker had a very exaggerated up-and-down motion to his or her steps, which Simms linked to alternating states of depression and buoyancy:

> The form of those so affected is quite in accordance with the up and down or undulatory appearance of the walk. Alternately you will find them in high spirits, full of hope and jubilant; again in deep depression, soon to rise into the opposite extreme. Hence the life of the plunger is one of fear and dread, hope and joy. His countenance most truthfully indicates this. Amid deep lines of sorrow and foreboding, may easily be perceived the laughing wrinkles round the eyes, and the traces of the cheerful smile that often plays around the mouth, and sets the chin so cheerily in harmony with the mobile lips. Almost in every instance the plunger will be found possessed of warm affection, but subject to deep depression on any want of affectionate reciprocation of the loving emotions.[59]

Even in the standard textbooks of psychiatry of the day, such as those of the Munich clinical psychiatrist Emil Kraepelin (1896), unnatural posture is a defining moment for mental illness. But these postures may be an indication of earlier evolutionary development with "attitudes of crouching like a beast without moving, standing or sitting in fixed poses which had an insane or delusional significance. . . ."[60] Thus the frozen catatonic posture is unnatural not only because it is frozen and unmoving over time but also because the positions themselves are pathological—i.e., the patients do not "stand up straight."

Inheritance is the key for such theories of posture. The model for the nineteenth century was evolutionary biology with a Lamarckian assumption about the inheritance of acquired characteristics. These alterations in posture were read as positive (if they were seen to be an increase in efficiency) or negative (if they were read as potentially a throwback to earlier, inefficient states of posture). Meanwhile, the eugenist Francis Galton (1869) postulated the existence of a "bell curve" with a "normal" distribution of positive and negative qualities that are bound to inheritance.[61] He created this in analogy to the "normal" distribution of height. While he began his categories of "genius" with "the judges of England between 1660 and 1865,"[62] he concluded with an appendix on oarsmen and wrestlers of the north country.[63] It is also evident that Galton, at least, saw the ability at sports to be a form of "genius" because of its inheritability. The eugenists thereafter "probed participants' physical and mental health by measuring posture and strength, peering into eyes, ears, and throats."[64] A military notion of posture and the plumb line is inherent in their understanding of bodily perfection.

The widely read Canadian physician and eugenist B. G. Jefferis defined this perfect posture at the close of the nineteenth century as the antithesis of illness and moral decay: "The following is said to be a correct posture for walking: Head erect: not too rigid; chin in, shoulders back. Permit no unnecessary motion about the thighs. Do not lean over to one side in walking, standing or sitting; the practice in walking, standing or sitting. The practice is not only ungraceful but deforming and therefore unhealthful."[65]

Jefferis's contemporaries in very different arenas also resorted to this idea of posture. In 1839, the French singer François Delsarte created a system of bodily training, which quickly became the dominant manner of training the body in every aspect of the public sphere. Delsarte saw the emotions as natural, claiming that every emotion had an expression and posture. He placed the ideal posture as "standing firm on both legs."[66]

The Victorian singing teacher George Copland, addressing gifted amateurs, suggests that they "stand up straight, and keep the shoulders well back, as this gives the lungs more room to properly expand. . . . There need be no stiffness in the attitude."[67] The singing master Francesco Lamperti (1813–1892) illustrates as late as 1921 that "the pupil should hold himself erect, with the chest expanded and the shoulders easy—in a word—in the position of a soldier."[68] The line between health and posture seems clear; between art and posture is equally evident in the time, as the aesthetic defines the human, while the grotesque and deformed denies the very essence of humanness.

Poor posture returns us to the very notion of what is human. H. G. Wells's *The Island of Doctor Moreau* (1896) presents the horrors of Moreau's experiments that merged animals with humans in terms of the erect posture of the offspring: "I could see the Thing rather more distinctly. It was no animal for it stood erect."[69] Over time they become more primitive, "and they walked erect with an increasing difficulty."[70] Yet "the dwindling shreds of the humanity still startled me every now and then a momentary recrudescence of speech, perhaps an unexpected dexterity of the fore feet, a pitiful attempt to walk erect."[71] They are experimental throwbacks into the world before Homo sapiens yet created by the very mind of the Homo sapiens. Wells's critique relies on the illusion of human progress and the malleability of posture as well as character: "a living being may . . . be regarded as raw material, as something plastic, something that may be shaped and altered, . . . and the organism as a whole developed far beyond its apparent possibilities. We overlook this collateral factor, and so too much of our modern morality becomes mere subservience to natural selection."[72] Posture may be changed, but there is always the anxiety of degeneration, of a "morbid deviation from the norm" (to use B. A. Morel's classic formulation from mid-century), from being an upright, erect human being devolving into some one or Thing that does not stand up straight.

H. G. Well's "Thing" is not quite human and therefore has not the erect posture that defines what is imagined to be the civilized being. Class as well as race are implicated in individuals with primitive posture, yet the idea that the lower classes are like more primitive animals seems never to quite vanish, as an essay in the *Lancet* noted in 1922:

> Some primitive races who have the squatting habit, and even many country people at home, keep the knees and back bent and have a carriage and gait not much better than that of the higher apes. As a

> general rule, the more highly civilised the people the better is the carriage, but a perfectly erect carriage cannot be attained without drill.[73]

This observation called forth a response by another physician who claimed that the lower class actually enjoyed the "all fours" position.[74]

The medicalization of working-class and middle-class fashion impacted on posture, from the training of women to more efficient work to middle-class use of corseting:

> . . . charwomen do not enjoy the "all fours" position, for they do not adopt it but merely a pseudo-quadruped attitude-viz., on the hands and knees, principally the latter, so that the hands may be freer for work—and that is the source of most of their troubles, the pads which they should wear being either missing or insufficient. Otherwise their work is very healthy, and the source of the popular objection to it is rather the stress put upon the pride than upon the back. Young girls in cookery schools, too, are now so full of the pride of the erect posture and of that lofty atmosphere to which their emotions have raised them that who dare mention to them such a lowly attitude as the "all fours" position, much less their adoption of it! Corsets, too, probably interfere.[75]

The anti-corseting literature is full of comments on the poor posture that results from corseting, forgetting that the corset was not merely a fashion item but was also a primary means of reforming the body of those suffering from poor posture, whether the result of rickets or poor education.[76]

In 1888, the Rational Dress Society in London protested in an editorial note in the opening number of its *Gazette* "against the introduction of any fashion in dress that either deforms the figure, impedes the movements of the body, or in any way tends to injure the health."[77] Posture was natural; all corseting caused deformation of posture and gait. The medical literature against corseting was extensive and argued that corseting deformed posture, bracketing the fact that corsets were also a standard means of treatment for scoliosis and hernia. An exchange in 1909–1910 between two British physicians in the *Lancet* about the dangers of corseting begins when the Wimpole Street physician Heather Bigg writes that "women have found by centuries of accumulated experience that corsets are to them structurally indispensable, whilst modern science has also shown that they are physiologically beneficial."[78] Cecil E. Fish responds quickly condemning the very idea that the corset may have beneficial results to posture; "If the erect posture demands it, then we should be wise to put our babies into stays soon they begin to toddle. God forbid it."[79] Bigg's response to this is of interest as it argues that erect posture may indeed be the cause of a wide range of aliments. Evolutionary medicine in its first epoch (it returns in the close of the twentieth century) seems to be able to divine the essential nature of human posture—and it is not upright:

> In writing on corsets some few years since I pointed this out, and, taking a mechanical or morphological view of the body, I explained it by the fact that man is built for a quadruped and not for an erect position, and that therefore neither his peritoneal slings nor his abdominal walls are adequate to resist the persistent drag of gravity upon his abdominal viscera. I also opined that in all likelihood the abdominal walls were by evolution strengthening, and it would appear from Mr. Arbuthnot Lane's observations than the peritoneal slings are tending also to strengthen in a similar way. And I advocated the use of corsets with the proper loin-band hold, because it appeared to me that they were in most instances positively necessary to combat the inherent structural disability under which mankind suffers when in the erect posture.[80]

The corset medically corrects a body damaged by its evolution to upright posture.

Speculations about the nature of correct and corrected gait and posture were the focus of the new science of photography, which was seen to provide empirical nature about how one walked or stood. Eadweard J. Muybridge attempted empirically to clarify these questions by using sequential photography to document human gait across class, "race," and disability in his photographic project on human and animal locomotion between 1883 and 1886. While indebted to the French chronophotographer Étienne-Jules Marey, Muybridge's work provided the first empirical evidence of human movement in space and time and set claims for all subsequent use of images to document posture. Indeed, it was Marey's photographic work that would inspire the first scientific study of human gait in Braune and Fischer's detailed atlas of military posture of 1889.

By the mid-twentieth century, "postural health" is defined as efficiency illustrated by normative images of the healthy and unhealthy body within medicine. Good posture is "important for proper functioning of the body and contributes to good appearance. Proper alignment of the body parts promotes efficiency of movement and endurance. The person who has good posture and who moves gracefully projects poise, confidence, and dignity."[81] It reflects character as well as health and beauty, as "faulty posture" is "unattractive." Good posture demands a postural education and constant self-correction to stand up straight:

> Head is held erect, not turned or tilted to one side.
> Shoulders are level.
> Arms hang easily at the sides with the palms of the hands toward the body.
> Hips are level, with the weight of the body borne equally by both legs.
> Kneecaps face straight ahead.
> Feet point straight ahead or toe out slightly.
> In other words, they may be parallel, or the feet may be about 1 inch further apart in front than at the heels.
> The weight of the body is carried toward the outer sides of the feet, and evenly balanced between the heel and the forefoot.
> Stand in front of a mirror and check to see that feet and knees are in good position, and that hips and shoulders are level. Make a habit of standing in a good position, with weight borne evenly on both feet. Good posture must be built from the feet up. If the feet and knees are in good position, there is a better chance that the rest of the body will line up properly. [82]

The "disabled" body is thus seen as having poor posture that demands correction in order to be healthy. This has its roots in the Enlightenment notion of retraining or repairing bad posture. The idea of an efficient posture that is part of an evolutionary pattern that leads to an ideal military body demands correction of disabled bodies or, in terms of the model of evolutionary development that defines posture as the first principle, extinction. Disability is thus to be found, as we shall see, as defined by poor posture within a wide range of categories, including gender and race.[83]

By the twentieth century, functional definitions of posture come to dominate the debate about posture, at least within medicine. Little attention is given to its origin. The Posture Committee of American Academy of Orthopedic Surgeons in 1947 defined posture as "the relative arrangement of the parts of the body," making a distinction between

> good posture: "the state of muscular and skeletal balance which protects the supporting structures of the body against injury or progressive deformity irrespective of the attitude in which these structures are working or resting" and poor posture as "a faulty relationship of the various parts of the body which produce increased strain on the supporting structures and in which there is less efficient balance of the body over its base of support."[84]

This is clearly the ideology that dominates Braune and Fischer's work on military posture in 1889 and becomes the officially accepted medical notion so that a standard textbook of the late twentieth century can define posture as a "position or attitude of the body; the relative arrangement of body parts for a specific activity; a characteristic manner of bearing one's body."[85] The idea of the functional efficiency inherent in the military model never vanishes, but thinkers such as Moshe Feldenkrais at mid-century argue that such postural "health" is not determined by an "ideal" body. Even severely disabled bodies can achieve postural efficiency: "Proper posture is such . . . that the movement is performed with the minimum of work, i.e., with the maximum of efficiency."[86] Efficiency is a Fordist concept, which reflects the fascination in the 1920s with time and motion studies such as those by Frank B. and Lillian Gilbreth as well as Frederick Winslow Taylor; it is the appropriate effort expended in the realm of work to accomplish a task.[87] This defines good posture in the translation of a military concept to the industrial world.

National Posture; Racial Posture

The idea of a political posture is, in the nineteenth century, closely associated with German nationalism rather than British eugenics, Galton's creation. "Turnvater Jahn" (Friedrich Ludwig Jahn [1778–1852]) did more than any other single individual to make bodily discipline a formal constituent part of German national identity. After absorbing the teachings of physicians such as Karl Basedow and Guts Muths, Jahn took gymnastics a step further, making popular gymnastics the cornerstone of an organic German nationalism that included mind, body, and politics. But there had been a longstanding claim that such notions of posture were social or cultural rather than biological. As early as the English physician John Bulwer's 1650 *Anthropometamorphosis: Man Transform'd, or the Artificial Changeling. Historically presented, in the mad and cruel Gallantry, foolish Bravery, ridiculous Beauty, filthy Fineness, and loathesome Loveliness of most Nations, fashioning & altering their Bodies from the Mould intended by Nature. With a Vindication of the Regular Beauty and Honesty of Nature, and an Appendix of the Pedigree of the English Gallant,* national bodies were seen to be based on cultural assumptions.[88] (Bulwer's work is an attack on fashion and change with clear political overtones of the day.) The French had a different posture than the Scots, and the English were different from everyone else. Certain nations exhibited acceptable posture; others idiosyncratic posture, which was to be condemned.

The idea that national characteristics of posture come to be understood as biological is nowhere better illustrated than in the work of Bulwer's contemporary Robert Burton, in his *Anatomy of Melancholy* (1621), which echoes such views and cites at least one group in terms of their posture. Burton writes of the "pace" of the Jews, as well as "their voice, . . . gesture, [and] looks," as a sign of "their conditions and infirmities."[89] Johann Jakob Schudt, the seventeenth-century German Orientalist, commented on the "crooked feet" of the Jews among other signs of their physical inferiority.[90] Difference in posture defines the Jew, but this difference may or may not be "racial" in its origin. Indeed, to paraphrase Burton, it may be the result of their oppressive lives and the illnesses that result from them.

What is folkloric (and Burton is not quite medical science) in the seventeenth century becomes part of the science of race in the nineteenth century. As early as 1804, in Joseph Rohrer's study of the Jews in the Austrian monarchy, the weak constitution of the Jew and its public sign, "weak feet," were cited as "the reason that the majority of Jews called into military service were released, because the majority of Jewish soldiers spent more time in the military hospitals than in military service." This link of the weak feet of the Jews and their inability to be full citizens (at a time when citizenship was being extended piecemeal to the Jews) was for Rohrer merely one further sign of the inherent, intrinsic difference of the Jews. Thus Balduin Groller can claim that the overwhelming evidence is that "the physical composition" of both Eastern and Western Jews "is not normal."[91] Groller cites the statistical records of a Russian military doctor on the prevalence of Jewish degeneracy: the average size of an adult Jew is 162.7 centimeters versus 165 to 170 centimeters for a non-Jew; Jews have less developed chest bones and musculature, including a 60 percent smaller chest size when compared to the norm; Jews suffer from bad posture as well as a greater susceptibility to tuberculosis, skin diseases, eye infections, myopia, and nervous and psychological disorders; and, finally, they have a greater incidence of hernia.[92] It is of little surprise that among the earliest medical specialists in the rather new field of orthopedics dealing with posture are two mid-nineteenth-century Jewish orthopedists in Berlin, Moritz Michael Eulenburg (1811–1887) and Heimann-Wolff Berend (1809–1873), who was the first to use anesthesia for surgery in Berlin. The latter also made early use of patient photographs to document and publicize the treatment of his patients.[93] Berend and Eulenburg were heavily influenced by the Swedish system of medical gymnastics developed by Pehr Henrik Ling, which was to reform posture and restore health through directed exercises. Bodies, even those of the Jews, were infinitely adaptable at least through medical intervention.

By the turn of the twentieth century, Jews, too, accept the notion of bad posture as a sign of their maladaptation into the modern world. Max Nordau, the most important figure in early Zionism after Theodor Herzl, in his opening speech at the Second Zionist Congress in Basel on August 28, 1898, invented one of Zionism's most famous, most fraught, and most challenging ideals: the "muscle Jew." His essay on "Muskeljudentum," often translated, "A Jewry of Muscle," which he originally gave as a dedicatory speech for the opening of yet another Jewish gymnastic club in 1903, condemned the "degenerate modernity" that he earlier saw defining the modern world:

> Unreal, too, are the studied postures, by assuming which the inmates are enabled to reproduce on their faces the light effects of Rembrandt or Schalcken. Everything in these houses aims at exciting the nerves and dazzling the senses.[94]

By the early twentieth century, he sees this as a maladaptation of the Jews: "The Jews' terrible posture does not come from any natural trait. It is but the result of a lack of psychical education. In this way, there is not really a difference between Jew and Aryan."[95] Nordau stated in 1903 that:

> I said: "We must once again think of creating a Jewry of muscle." . . . Once again! For history is our witness that such a Jewry once existed. There is no shame to admitting this need: Our new muscle Jews [*Muskeljuden*] have not yet regained the heroism of their forefathers . . . to take part in battles and compete with the trained Hellenic athletes and strong northern barbarians. But morally speaking, we are better off today than yesterday, for the old Jewish circus performers of yore were ashamed of their Judaism and sought, by way of a surgical pinch, to hide the sign of their religious affiliation . . . while today, the members of Bar Kochba proudly and freely proclaim their Jewishness.[96]

Simon Bar Kochba, of course, was the warrior who led the Jews in their failed revolt against the Romans in 132 CE, after whom the sporting societies were named. The Jews are the sick *men* of Europe:

> Zionist societies use every effort that the members and the Jewish masses in general may know the history of their nation, and become acquainted with the sacred and profane literature in the Hebrew tongue. They teach the Jews to hold their heads high, to be proud of

> their descent, and to despise the anti-Semitic lies . . . they care, in the measure of their strength, for the amelioration of the hygiene of the Jewish proletariat, for its economic improvement by means of association and solidarity, for well directed education of children, and for the instruction of women . . . they preach the duty of leading a faultless, spiritual life, the rejection of crude materialism, into which the assimilation Jews, on account of the want of a worthy ideal, are only too apt to sink, and strict self-control in word and deed. They found athletic societies in order to promote the long neglected physical development of the rising generation.[97]

In speaking about the newly established Jewish National Fund during the Fifth Zionist Congress in Basel in 1901, Nordau argued:

> The physical elevation of the Jewish people is a money question. If the [majority] of Jews were in a good position it would not be necessary to waste words on their physical improvement . . . look at the Jewish families who for the past three generations have been men of wealth! Compare these stately horsemen, these first rate fighters, these stylist dancers, these prize-winning gymnasts and swimmers, compare their robust bodies with the emaciated and coughed-racked frames of the Eastern ghettos. Then you will immediately form an idea of the means required for the physical amelioration of the Jewish race. . . . The mass has neither the time nor the means for gymnastics and sports. If we offer them any hygienic suggestions it must be such that cost nothing.[98]

This biological notion of regeneration of good posture is very much in line with Theodor Herzl's views on adaption and mal-adaptation: "Education can be achieved only through shock treatment. Darwin's theory of imitation [*Darwinsche Mimikry*] will be validated. The Jews will adapt. They are like seals that have been thrown back into the water by an accident of nature . . . if they return to dry land and manage to stay there for a few generations, their fins will change back into legs."[99] And one can add, they will "stand up straight." As Paul Higate observed: "Only by providing a 'previously emasculated Central European Jewry with an honorable and manly posture' did Theodor Herzl believe the goal of the regeneration of a Jewish state could be achieved."[100] But this was not only an ideal. The self-consciously Jewish strongman Siegmund né Zishe Breitbart (1883–1925) became the image of the "new muscle Jew" in Herzl's Vienna and beyond:

> A human being of supernatural powers. Breitbart. He bends steel as if it were soft rubber, bites through chains as though they were tender meat, drives nails into thick wood with his bare fist. . . . A bridge loaded with hundreds of kilograms of concrete block is lowered onto his gigantic body, and the blocks are pounded with hammers. . . .[101]

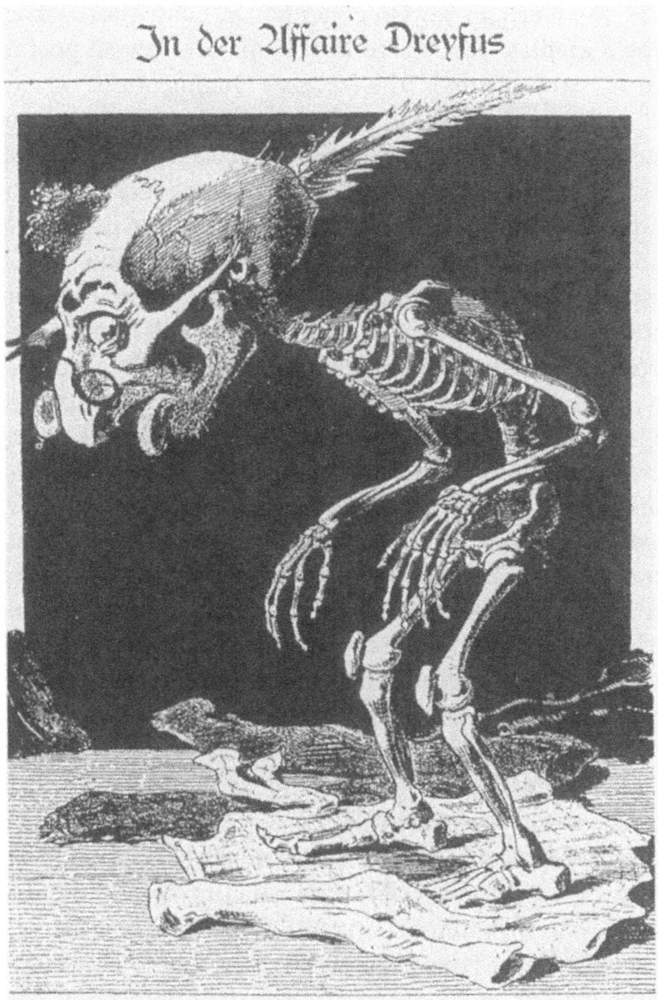

Figure 3.7. The fantasy of Jewish posture in the first age of the X-ray. From the anti-Semitic Viennese periodical *Kikiriki* during the Dreyfus affair. Reproduced in Eduard Fuchs, *Die Juden in der Karikatur: ein Beitrag zur Kulturgeschichte* (München: Eduard Langen, 1921), 203.

Costuming himself as Bar Kochba, he came to represent the new muscle Jew as pseudo-military figure. Sport becomes the means, as it was in the nineteenth century German national movement to regenerate not only a healthy body but also a healthy mind. Through such twentieth century transformation the Jew regains a pride in being Jewish through the newly revitalized Jewish body.

In 1908, the German-Jewish eugenist Dr. Elias Auerbach of Berlin undertook a medical rebuttal to the claims of a Jewish postural inferiority, in an essay entitled "The Military Qualifications of the Jew," of the "fact" of the predisposition of the Jew for certain disabilities which precluded him from military service.[102] Auerbach begins by attempting to "correct" the statistics, which claimed that for every 1,000 Christians in the population there were 11.61 soldiers, but for 1,000 Jews in the population there were only 4.92 soldiers. His correction (based on the greater proportion of Jews entering the military who were volunteers and, therefore, did not appear in the statistics) still finds that a significant portion of Jewish soldiers were unfit for service (according to his revised statistics, of every 1,000 Christians there were 10.66 soldiers; of 1,000 Jews, 7.76). He accepts the physical differences of the Jew as a given but questions whether there is a substantive reason that these anomalies should prevent the Jew from serving in the military. He advocates the only true solution that will make the Jews of equal value as citizens: the introduction of "sport" and the resultant reshaping of the Jewish body. In 1909, Max Zirker argued in the *Jewish Gymnastics Journal* that the Jewish people must develop a "class of farmers" who can till the ground, something that will counterbalance their "mostly intellectual work." As such, they will develop the bones, musculature, and posture necessary for serving in the military and becoming national citizens able to defend a future homeland, while also honing their intellectual prowess and "mental hygiene."[103]

These maladaptations are forms of mental illness, as the Italian psychiatrist Enrico Morselli observed when he coined the diagnostic category of "dysmorphophobia" in 1891. Dysmorphophobia is, according to Morselli, the fact that patients stressed their own fixed physiognomy of the patient as the source of their unhappiness. He described the patients' fixation on specific qualities of that body: the low and mashed forehead, the absurd nose, and the bandy legs. Bad posture and badly formed bodies are the origin of mental illness.

This view of the pathological meaning of poor posture is found through the defenses of the Jews with the rise of racial anti-Semitism at the close of the nineteenth century. Anatole Leroy-Beaulieu, in his 1893 "defense" of the Jews, notes that the Jews are characterized by the predominance of the nervous system over the muscular system: "too little muscles; too much nerves, il est tout nerfs [he is all nerves]." The Jew is all nerves because of his "oriental origin" and his sedentary life.[104] Joseph Pennell, the illustrator and friend of James McNeil Whistler, in a small book on *The Jew at Home* (serialized in the *London Illustrated News* at the same time) states more or less the same problem among Russian Jews:

> The Jew naturally is not physically weaker than the peasant. As a soldier, when he is made to stand up straight, he is as fine a man as any other Russian, with the exception that he cannot march as well, but becomes quickly footsore. This is because he never takes any exercise. . . .[105]

Every view of the Jew's body sees bad posture at its core reflecting, in one way or another, the character of the Jew.

At the same moment, the anti-Semites are making the same argument/drawing the same connection. In 1893, the German physician-writer Oskar Panizza, in his depiction of the Jewish body, observed that the Jew's body language was clearly marked:

> When he walked, Itzig always raised both thighs almost to his midrift so that he bore some resemblance to a stork. At the same time he lowered his head deeply into his breast-plated tie and stared at the ground.—Similar disturbances can be noted in people with spinal diseases. However, Itzig did not have a spinal disease, for he was young and in good condition.[106]

The Jew looks as if he is diseased, but it is not the stigmata of degeneracy that the observer is seeing, but the Jew's natural stance. The anthropologist Hans F. K. Günther published pictures of "typical Jewish posture"; as well as popularizing *Rassenkunde* [race science] and the idea of Nordic supremacy, he contributed to the problem of how to identify Jews by describing such pathological but "typical Jewish posture."[107] This view becomes the touchstone for Nazi racial politics in a pragmatic manner. When Heinrich Himmler's "race office" develops criteria to sort "racially acceptable" from "unacceptable" individuals among the occupied nations of Europe after 1941, for inclusion as Aryans "erect bearing" trumped all other criteria. As Peter Longreich noted in his biography of Himmler, this would have excluded Himmler from inclusion as "racially acceptable" given his poor posture.[108]

Scholars of the body politics of Stalinist Russia in the 1930s have pointed out that the cultural and public discourse of the time was marked by the rhetoric of reforging (*perekovka*) human beings. In spite of this culture's Marxist emphasis on the supremacy of the economic and social environment for human formation, the concept of reforging was paradoxically linked to the notion of biological change within an organism. Various Jewish writers, such as children's book writer Lev Kassil, made attempts to demonstrate the success of such a reforging of the body and soul as exhibited in many Russian and Jewish characters in the writing of the 1930s. The human body's biological essence was viewed as a product of the forces of nature against which remedies had to be found. As Mikhail Zoshchenko's diaries attest, Max Nordau's turn-of-the century concept of degeneration continued to be influential among the generation of the 1930s, and the question of overcoming degeneration was of great importance to this generation.[109] Learning to stand up straight was a key to this in shaping the new Soviet Man (as well as the new Fascist Man and the new Zionist Man), as much as sexual identity as George Mosse argued.[110] The Marxist philosopher Ernst Bloch "saw the upright gait as a moral orthopedics of human dignity, as strengthening the backbone against humiliation, dependency, and subjugation."[111] Bloch reads upright gait as a political act and sees it as standing behind Marx's demand "to overthrow all relations in which man is a degraded, enslaved, abandoned, or despised being." He observed that "the claim to the upright gait was within all rebellions; otherwise there would not be uprisings. The very word uprising means that one makes one's way out of one's horizontal, dejected, or kneeling position into an upright one."[112] In other words, stand up straight.

National and Political Posture in Asia

How we stand defines who we are in the eye of the beholder but also in our own bodily sense. But all of these claims were also part of a Western attempt to use posture (and the means of altering it) as the litmus test for the healthy modern body of the perfect citizen. Focusing on the centrality of posture in two oddly linked moments of modern thought—modern Zionist thought and Nationalism in early-twentieth-century China—in terms of bodily reform, all of the earlier Western claims about posture (and the body of the "sick Jew" as well as the "sick *man* of Asia") brings all of the earlier debates together to reform unhealthy posture.

In Asia "bad" posture was "good" posture, as "Chinese posture also reflects social relationships: rounded shoulders characterize the bow, which is an expression of humility before superiors, and in the case of athletes, also before audiences."[113] As Western medicine came into China during the nineteenth century, this notion of posture defined the "sick man of Asia," as Larissa N. Heinrich discusses in her

The Afterlife of Images: Translating the Pathological Body between China and the West (2008). But being "sick" was also seen as a reflex of the degenerate culture of late Imperial China: "Few nations make use of so many compliments as the Chinese. Bowing, kneeling, and prostrating themselves are the different grades of the respect they show toward each other."[114] Such social posture quickly came to be a sign of the degeneracy of Chinese culture in the creation of sick bodies:

> The myriads of beggars also go in for voluntary deformation crawling on their knees till they cannot assume an upright posture; welcoming and encouraging an ulcer or a skin disease or a blind eye until the utmost possible deformity and condition of filth are attained. When no better result can be accomplished, something may always be done with paint and plasters, and a very good imitation of the real thing produced.[115]

Degeneracy was the key[116] but it was a socially-created degeneracy, and was so seen at least by the most radical writer of the time Lu Xun who wrote in 1918: "The world is going to the dogs. Men are growing more degenerate every day. The country is faced with ruin!' such laments have been heard in China since time immemorial. But 'degeneracy' varies from age to age. It used to mean one thing, now it means another."[117]

Posture remained tied in with the question of pride and confidence, so to "lift one's head" is not only what the Chinese nation should do metaphorically on the global stage, but also what the Chinese people literally must do to march into "modernity." Confidence as with Max Nordau and the Zionist is tied to notions of pride in a new Chinese body. Being "spineless" and "slouching" is not only a problem of the Chinese nation on the political stage but also a problem of the people's bodies. There are scattered references to this kind of argument in 1920s journals and magazines (especially in etiquette manuals which tell one how to dress, eat, meet and greet, and walk—complete with illustrations—that have this nationalist rhetoric to varying degrees). Even Zhang Jingsheng, the Shanghai commentator known as "Dr. Sex," touches upon the question of sitting/standing up straight in his "aesthetic utopia"; there is one universal, "aesthetic" way of sitting/standing that must be adopted by all.[118] There is a counter-discourse to this in the "modernist" loafer like Lin Yutang who in his *Importance of Living* (1937) observes that there is nothing wrong with loafing, lying around—that all this talk of how people should sit, stand and walk is oppressive, enforcing conformity, turning everyone into efficient soldiers and machines with no individual character.[119]

It is of little surprise that just as the Jews were reforming their bodies as part of a new national ideology of Jewish identity, revolutionary China came to the same conclusion: reform posture and you reform the system. Social Darwinism entered China with modernization. Yan Fu was one of the principal figures to introduce Darwin's natural selection, to China in the late nineteenth century.[120] Central to this was the notion of adaptability, and posture is central to this idea. Chen Duxiu, the cofounder of the Chinese Communist Party in 1921, made this idea part of the ideology of Chinese communism, especially in his periodical *New Youth*. In 1915 he complained that

> Whenever I look at our educated youth, I see that they have not the strength to catch a chicken, nor mentally the courage of an ordinary man. With pale faces and slender waists, seductive as young ladies, timorous of cold and chary of heat, weak as invalids—if the people of our country are as feeble as this in body and mind how will they be able to shoulder burdens and go far?[121]

As the historian Frank Dikötter noted:

> A strict upright posture was prescribed to youngster under the Guomindang's New Life Movement in the 1930s, and today it is still the characteristic way in which young party members are portrayed in communist propaganda. On the other hand a bearing which denoted indolence was attached and every effort was made to correct slovenly gestures: these became the marks of physical degeneration and spiritual decay. . . . After 1900 there was an emphasis on physical training and martial vigour, and this ranged from Luo Zhenyu's recommendation to turn Confucian temples into physical training centres to Mao Zedong's writings on physical exercise.[122]

While Mao Tse-tung's youthful work on combating the degeneracy of Chinese society and the body was in the time truly marginal, it can serve as a model for the arguments about reforming posture that paralleled the Zionist case.[123] His "A Study of Physical Education" which was an essay published in April 1917 (in *Hsin ching-nein*) argues in the model of Turnvater Jahn that sick minds inhabit sick bodies: "Those whose bodies are small and frail are flippant in their behaviour. Those whose skin is flabby are soft and dull in will. Thus does the body influence the mind."[124] And the ill mind of the Chinese is reflected in their politics.

Yet Mao's argument is very much post-Darwinian:

> Because man is an animal, movement is most important for him. And because he is a rational animal, his movements must have a reason. But why is movement deserving of esteem? Why is rational movement deserving of esteem? To say that movement helps in earning a living is trivial. To say that movement protects the nation is lofty. Yet neither is the basic reason. The object of movement is simply to preserve our life and gladden our hearts." . . . Physical education not only strengthens the body but also enhances our knowledge. There is a saying: Civilize the mind and make savage the body. This is an apt saying. In order to civilize the mind one must first make savage the body. If the body is made savage, then the civilized mind will follow. Knowledge consists in knowing the things in the world, and in discerning their laws. In this matter we must rely on our body, because direct observation depends on the ears and eyes, and reflection depends on the brain. The ears and eyes, as well as the brain, may be considered parts of the body. When the body is perfect, then knowledge is also perfect.[125]

The end result is the creation of the upright posture advocated for the military from the seventeenth century:

> Our nation is wanting in strength. The military spirit has not been encouraged; the physical condition of the population deteriorates daily. This is an extremely disturbing phenomenon. The promoters of physical education have not grasped the essence of the problem, and therefore, their efforts, though prolonged, have not been effective. If this state continues, our weakness will increase further. To attain our goals and to make our influence felt are external matters, results. The development of our physical strength is an internal matter, a cause. If our bodies are not strong we will be afraid as soon as we see enemy soldiers, and then how can we attain our goals and make ourselves respected? Strength depends on drill, and drill depends on self-awareness.[126]

The military model is Darwinian but also revolutionary.

The link to the West is clearly made in Mao's text: "East and West differ in their interpretations of it. Chuang Tzu followed the example of the cook, Confucius drew on the lesson of the archer and the charioteer. In Germany, Physical Education has gained the greatest popularity. Fencing has spread all over the country."[127] This link has been overlooked because it seems quite an offhanded remark. Fencing as a popular sport? Rather dueling! And it is dueling that historically is the litmus test in late-nineteenth-century German for answering the question of Jewish masculinity and identity in bourgeois society. During the nineteenth century, Jewish students were automatically admitted to the general fraternity systems in Germany, which were dueling societies. There one learned the rules of social behavior and of physical deportment. Saber fencing had its own specific posture. Many acculturated Jews, such as Theodor Herzl "relished the test and adventure of the duel, the so-called *Mensur*, which was considered manly and edifying."[128] Students challenged each other to duels as a matter of course, without any real need for insults to be exchanged; being challenged was a process of social selection. "Without exclusivity—no corporation," was the code of the fraternities as late as 1912.[129] By then, Jews had been expelled from the general fraternity system, and Jewish dueling fraternities sprang up. Being *satisfaktionsfähig* (worthy of satisfaction), meant members of these fraternities were seen as honorable equals and thus could be challenged to a duel. Marked on the duelist's scarred face and erect posture was his integration into German culture. This was the context in which the Jewish fraternities (most of which did not duel) sought to reconfigure the sickly Jewish body into what the early Zionist Max Nordau called the "new muscle Jew." The Jewish fraternity organization stated in 1902 that "it desires the physical education of its members in order to collaborate in the physical regeneration of the Jewish people."[130] For some Jews, a duel marked the socially healthy individual.

Mao's demand in 1916 was for the ideology, if not the technique of fencing, so that the Chinese body would become "real Chinese" and not mere simulacra:

> At present, most people overemphasize knowledge. During the years of middle school, the development of the body is not yet completed. Since today the factors favouring physical development are few, and those deterring it numerous, won't physical development tend to cease? In the educational system of our country, required courses are as thick as the hairs on a cow. Even an adult with a tough, strong body could not stand it let alone those who have not reached adulthood, or those who are weak. Speculating on the intentions of the educators, one is led to wonder whether they did not design such an unwieldy curriculum in order to exhaust the students, to trample on their bodies and ruin their lives. . . . How stupid![131]

Mao's view may well have been impacted if indirectly by the role that Zionist thought had in the development of Nationalism in Asia. While there only a marginal presence of Zionist views in China, as Zhou Xun

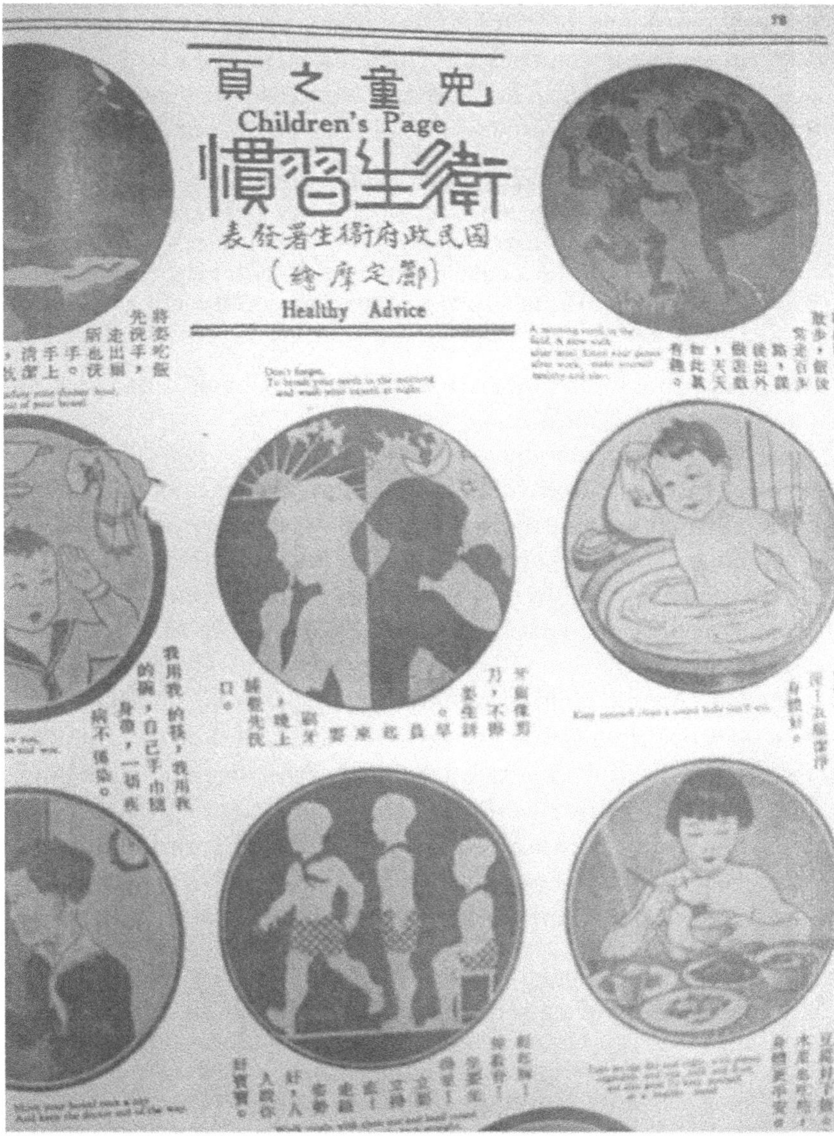

Figure 3.8. A page from a Republican Chinese guide for teachers, unpaged, undated (private collection).

has argued, it is clear that Max Nordau's views were widely circulated in the modernist reforms of Meiji Japan after 1868, where many Chinese thinkers had their first exposure to modernity and ideas of bodily reform.[132] Part of the struggle for the modern Chinese body had to do with the elimination of foot binding, now seen as an antiquated practice to control the bodies of women that typified Imperial China. In the United States, "Chinese-American ladies shoes" led to bad posture. Therefore, bad posture was not the result of foot binding but of being Chinese:

> But the other evil is equally bad and is especially almost exclusively a woman's danger. The foot is made too small and too high and is displaced forward. Its narrowness makes women unsteady in their gait like the Chinese. Their equilibrium is unstable. Its height is still worse. The sole is on an inclined plane as if the wearer constantly going down a mountain and how fatiguing that is let any one say after a trial.[133]

The bound foot leads women to walk "like the Chinese." Bad posture is a quality of the Chinese body.

Such views are not marginal in Chinese thought following the Xinhai Revolution that began with the Wuchang Uprising on October 10, 1911, and ended with the abdication of Emperor Puyi on February 12, 1912. The Nationalist government by the 1920s demanded in their educational system, as had Mao, healthy posture and beautiful children.[134] One pamphlet published by the Republican government Public Health Bureau teaches children how to stand up straight, how to sit, and how to walk. It is headed: "A good child must have correct posture." No degenerate bodies; only healthy posture for the new citizens of the new China.

Yet these "beautiful" children, a demand of the eugenics of the time, are not simply Chinese. Health and beauty can be found in the United States in the realm of posture well beyond the school classroom, and the counterpoint to the masculine history of posture comes to be found in the history of modern feminine beauty. As a historian of posture noted:

> Posture Queen Programs had their beginning in the Most Perfect Spine Contest of the American Chiropractic Association (1922–1930) at its 1927 convention. At the 1935 NCA Convention in Hollywood, California, the winner of the two-hundred-contestant event was known as Miss Perfection. Life-sized, entire body x-rays were displayed along with a parade of finalists in bathing suits and evenings gowns with low backs.[135]

Beauty (bathing suits), health (X-rays), and posture are not particularly American definitions of the healthy feminine—German and French sources of the nineteenth century point toward this as well—but the shift from the realm of the military to the realm of beauty represents the traditional universes of the masculine and the feminine bodies defined here by posture.[136] The entangled genealogies of posture are reflected in

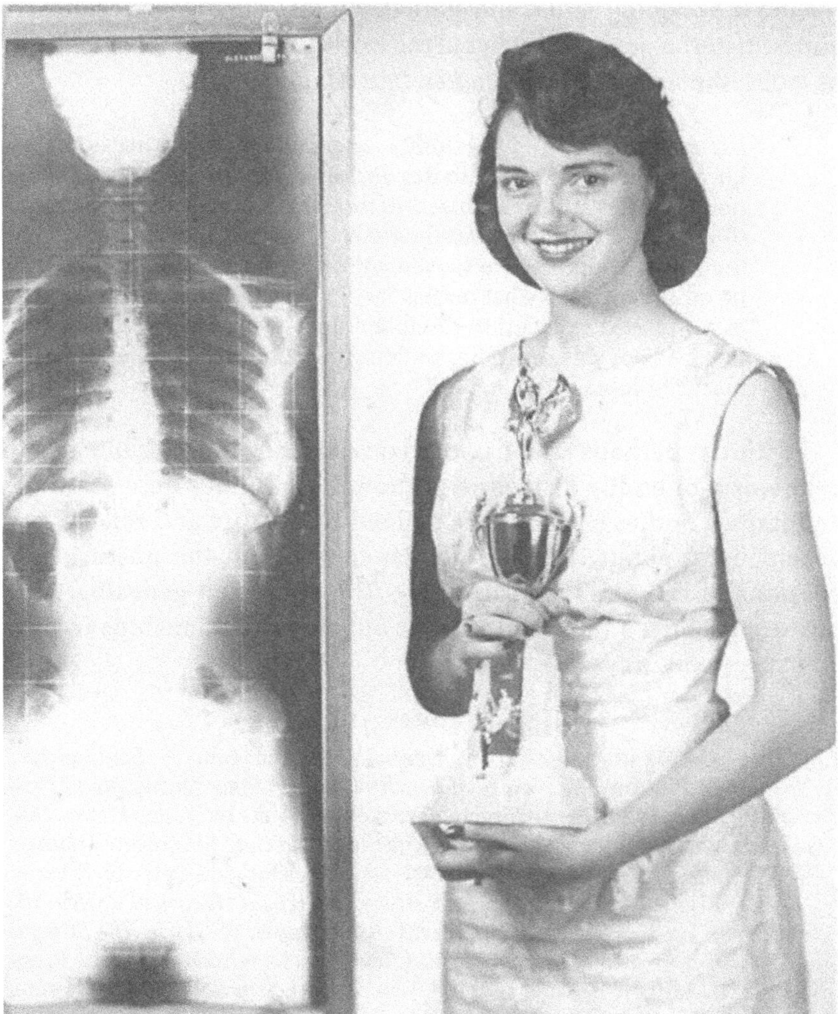

Figure 3.9. Miss Peggy Jackson of Hackneyville, Alabama, winner of the 1960 Annual Posture Queen Contest with her full spinal X-ray. From P. Reginald Hug, "Posture Queen Contests in Alabama," *Journal of Chiropractic Humanities* 15 (2008): 67–80.

virtually every discussion of the nature and form of the human—from race to gender, from pathology to beauty— it is, to use Donna Haraway's term, a "corporeal fetish" that mistakes "heterogeneous relationality for a fixed, seemingly objective thing." Of equal importance in studying the history of posture is the assumption that the specific use of posture "denies the ongoing action and work that it takes to sustain technoscientific material-semiotic bodies in the world."[137] It is a slippery concept, as Judith Butler observed in *Bodies That Matter:*

> . . . the materiality of the body . . . moved me into other domains. I tried to discipline myself to stay on the subject, but found that I could not fix bodies as simple objects of thought. Not only did bodies tend to indicate a world beyond themselves, but this movement beyond their own boundaries, a movement or boundary itself appeared to be quite central to what bodies "are." I kept losing track of the subject. I proved resistant to discipline. Inevitably, I began to consider that perhaps this resistance to fixing the subject was essential to the matter at hand.[138]

Posture is perhaps an index of that resistance to discipline in the very world of bodily discipline. It draws bright lines between male and female bodies seen as sites defined by posture and reflects the very debates about race and gender inherent in the posture discussions of the nineteenth century. The entangled genealogies of posture provide a means of teasing out these relationships in new and surprising ways.

Notes

1. The existing literature on the subject is limited: John A. Schumacher, *Human Posture: The Nature of Inquiry* (Albany: State University of New York Press, 1989); Bernd Jürgen Warneken and Anka Blashofer-Hrusa, eds., *Der aufrechte Gang. Zur Symbolik einer Körperhaltung.* (Tübingen: Tübinger Vereinigung für Volkskunde, 1990); David Yosifon and Peter N. Stearns, "The Rise and Fall of American Posture," *American Historical Review* 103 (1998): 1057–1095; Peter N. Stearns, *Battleground of Desire: The Struggle for Self-control in Modern America* (New York: New York University Press, 1999); Matthew B. Roller, *Dining Posture in Ancient Rome: Bodies, Values and Status* (Princeton, NJ: Princeton University Press, 2006).
2. Karen Barad, *Meeting the Universe Halfway: Quantum Physics and the Entanglement of Matter and Meaning.* (Durham: Duke University Press, 2002), here 390.
3. Ibid., 389.
4. All of these references are from the *Oxford English Dictionary*'s definition of "posture," http://www.oed.com.proxy.library.emory.edu/ (accessed November 7, 2013).
5. MacGregor Knox and Murray Williamson, eds. *The Dynamics of Military Revolution, 1300–2050* (Cambridge: Cambridge University Press, 2001), here 49.
6. S. J. Walker, "Arms and the Man: Constructing the Soldier in Jacques de Gheyn's 'Wapenhandelinghe'" *Nederlands Kunsthistorisch Jaarboek* 58 (2007/2008): 138–6.

7. Ben Jonson, *The Workes of Benjamin Jonson*. (London: Printed for Richard Meighen, 1640), here 38.
8. Immanuel Kant, "Idea for a Universal History with a Cosmopolitan Aim" In Allen Wood, trans., *The Cambridge Edition of the Works of Immanuel Kant: Anthropology, History and Education*, Günter Zöller and Robert B. Louden, eds. (Cambridge: Cambridge University Press, 2007).
9. Karl Gaulhofer, *Die Fusshaltung. Ein Beitrag zur Stilgeschichte der menschlichen Bewegung* (Kassel: Wissenschaftliche Gesellschaft für körperliche Erziehung, 1930), here 62.
10. William Hardy McNeill, *Keeping Together in Time: Dance and Drill in Human History* (Cambridge, MA: Harvard University Press, 1995), here 2.
11. Michel Foucault, *Discipline & Punish: The Birth of the Prison*, Alan Sheridan, trans. (New York: Vintage Books, 1995), here 135.
12. Ibid., 135.
13. Ibid., 135.
14. Ibid., 136.
15. Henry Hitchings, *Defining the World, The Extraordinary Story of Dr. Johnson's Dictionary* (New York: Farrar, Straus & Giroux, 2005), here 166.
16. Walter Scott, *The Waverly Novels*, 30 Vols. *Kenilworth*, Vol. 12. (London: Nimmo, 1893), here 359.
17. Christian Wilhelm Braune and Otto Fischer, *Über den Schwerpunkt des menschlichen Körpers mit Rücksicht auf die Ausrüstung des deutschen Infanteristen* (Leipzig: S. Hirzel, 1889), here 3–4. The English language reprint *On the Centre of Gravity of the Human Body as Related to the Equipment of the German Infantry Soldier* (Berlin; New York: Springer-Verlag, 1985). See also Christian Wilhelm Braune and Otto Fischer, *Der Gang des Menschen*. (Leipzig: B. G. Teubner, 1899). The English language reprint as *Human Mechanics* (Springfield, VA: Distributed by National Technical Information Service, 1963).
18. McNeill, *Keeping Together*, 1.
19. Braune and Fischer, *Über den Schwerpunkt des menschlichen Körpers*, here 6–7.
20. "Medicine: Posture Lady," *Time*, April 5, 1937. At http://www.time.com/time/magazine/article/0,9171,757573,00.html (accessed November 7, 2013).
21. Ibid.
22. C. Owen Lovejoy, "The Natural History of Human Gait and Posture: Part 1. Spine and Pelvis," *Gait & Posture* 21 (2005): 95–112, here p. 95; See C. Owen Lovejoy, "The Natural History of Human Gait and Posture: Part 2. Hip and Thigh," *Gait & Posture* 21 (2005): 113–124; C. Owen Lovejoy, "The Natural History of Human Gait and Posture: Part 3. The Knee," *Gait & Posture* 25 (2007): 325–341.
23. Ann Gibbons, "A New Kind of Ancestor: Ardipithecus Unveiled." *Science* 326, no. 5949 (October 2009): 36–40, here 36. See also the overviews by Carol V. Ward, "Early Hominin Posture and Locomotion: Where Do We Stand?" *Yearbook of Physical Anthropology* 45 (2002), 186–215; "The Evolution of Human Origins," *American Anthropologist* 105 (2003), 77–88. A popular introduction remains Jonathan Kingdon, *Lowly Origin: Where, When, and Why Our Ancestors First Stood Up* (Princeton, NJ: Princeton University Press, 2003).

24. T. D. White, et al., "Ardipithecus Ramidus and the Paleobiology of Early Hominids," *Science* 326, no. 5949 (October 1, 2009): 64–64, 75–86.
25. Sir Arthur Keith, *The Construction of Man's Family Tree.* (London: Watts and Co., 1934), here 15.
26. Marjorie O'Rourke Boyle, *Senses of Touch: Human Dignity and Deformity from Michelangelo to Calvin* (Boston: Brill Academic Pub, 1998), here 31–33.
27. All references are to Pavel Gregorić, "Plato's and Aristotle's Explanation of Human Posture," *RHIZAI* II.2 (2005), 183–196.
28. Aristotle, *De partibus animalium,* IV.10 686a 27–31.
29. Plato, *Timaeus,* 45a1, 91e-92a.
30. Plato, *Timaeus,* 90a2–b1.
31. William Heinemann, *Xenophon,* E. C. Marchant, trans., (Cambridge, MA: Harvard University Press, 1968), here 57–58.
32. Laertius Diogenes, *Diogenes Laertius: Lives of Eminent Philosophers,* 9 Vols., R. D. Hicks, trans., Loeb Classical Library (Cambridge, MA: Harvard University Press, 1925), here 40.
33. Johann Gottfried Herder, *Outlines of a Philosophy of the History of Man,* T. Churchill, trans. (London: J. Johnson, 1800), here 67–68.
34. Ibid., 49.
35. Ibid., 70.
36. (*Paradise Lost* VII, 506–15)
37. Immanuel Kant, *Universal History.*
38. Ibid., 17.
39. Karl Rosenkranz, *Aesthetik des Hässlichen* (Königsberg: Gebrüder Bornträger, 1853), here 51.
40. Ibid., 52.
41. Jean-Baptiste de Lamarck, *Philosophie zoologique, ou exposition des considérations relatives à l'histoire naturelle des animaux...* (Paris: Dentu, 1809), here 349.
42. Cited by Gustav Muskat, "Ist der Plattfuss eine Rasseneigentümlichket?" *Im Deutschen Reich* (1909), 354–58, here 354.
43. Robert J. Richards, *The Meaning of Evolution: The Morphological Construction and Ideological Reconstruction of Darwin's Theory* (Chicago: University of Chicago Press, 1993).
44. Robert Munro, *Prehistoric Problems, Being a Selection of Essays on the Evolution of Man and Other Controverted Problems in Anthropology and Archæology* (Edinburgh, London, W. Blackwood and sons, 1897).
45. Charles Darwin, *The Descent of Man, and Selection in Relation to Sex* (London: J. Murray, 1871), here 137–139.
46. Ibid., 137–139.
47. Friedrich Engels, *The Part Played by Labour in the Transition from Ape to Man* (Moscow: Progress Publishers, 1972), here 4.
48. Ibid.
49. G. H. Estabrooks, *Man The Mechanical Misfit.* (New York: Macmillan, 1941), here 96.
50. Mitchell Ash, "Wissenschaft und Politik als Ressourcen fur einander," in Rudiger vom Buch and Brigitte Kaderas, eds., *Wissenschaften und Wissenschaftspolitik. Bestandsaufnahme und Perspektiven der Forschung* (Stuttgart: Franz Steiner, 2002).

51. Klaus Theweleit, *Männerphantasien*. 2 Vols. (Frankfurt: Roter Stern, 2002), here 62.
52. Michael Hau, *The Cult of Health and Beauty in Germany: A Social History, 1890–1930* (Chicago: University of Chicago Press, 2003), here 157.
53. Peter Sloterdijk, *Weltfremdheit* (Erstausgabe. Suhrkamp Verlag, 1993), here 235.
54. C. O. Lovejoy, "Evolution of Human Walking." *Scientific American* 259, no. 5 (1988): 118–25, here 120.
55. Ibid., 120.
56. Angela Willey, "From Pair-Bonding to Polyamory: A Feminist Critique of Naturalizing Discourses on Monogamy and Non-Monogamy" (PhD Diss., Emory University, 2009).
57. Constance Malpas, "Jules Guerin Makes his Market: The Social Economy of Orthopaedic Medicine in Paris, 1825–45." In Willem de Blécourt, Cornelie Usborne, eds., *Cultural Approaches to the History of Medicine: Mediating Medicine in Early Modern and Modern Europe*, 187–213 (New York: Palgrave MacMillan, 2004).
58. Joseph Simms, *Physiognomy Illustrated: Or, Nature's Revelations of Character. A Description of the Mental, Moral, and Volitive Dispositions of Mankind, as Manifested in the Human Form and Countenance* (New York: Murray Hill Pub. Co., 1887), here 267.
59. Ibid., 397.
60. Anon., "The Stereotyped Attitudes and Postures of the Insane in Regard to Diagnosis and Prognosis." *The Lancet* 159, no. 4094 (February 1902): 465–466.
61. Francis Galton, *Hereditary Genius: An Inquiry into Its Laws and Consequences* (London: Macmillan, 1869), here 23.
62. Ibid., 55.
63. Ibid., 305.
64. Christine Rosen, *Preaching Eugenics: Religious Leaders and the American Eugenics Movement* (New York: Oxford University Press, 2004), here 113.
65. Benjamin Grant Jefferis and J. L. Nichols. *Searchlights on Health: Light on Dark Corners A Complete Sexual Science and a Guide to Purity and Physical Manhood, Advice To Maiden, Wife, And Mother, Love, Courtship, And Marriage* (Toronto: J.L. Nichols, 1894), here 34.
66. Robin Veder, "The Expressive Efficiencies of American Delsarte and Mensendieck Body Culture." *Modernism/modernity* 17, no. 4 (2010): 819–38.
67. George Copland, "Hints on Singing," *The Minim: A Musical Magazine for Everybody* 4, no. 43 (April 1897): 164–165, here 164–165.
68. Francesco Lamperti, *The Art of Singing*, J. C. Griffith, trans. and ed. (London: G. Schirmer, 1939), here 3.
69. H. G. Wells, *The Island of Dr. Moreau* (Garden City, NY: Garden City Publishing, 1896), here 83.
70. Ibid., 230.
71. Ibid., 233.
72. [H.G. Wells], "The Limits of Individual Plasticity," *The Saturday Review* (January 19, 1895), 89–90, here, 90.
73. Thompson, J. Knox, "The Erect Posture." *The Lancet* 199, no. 5136 (February 1922): 251, here 107.

74. Harry Campbell, "The Erect Posture." *The Lancet* 199, no. 5134 (January 1922): 154.
75. Knox, "Posture", 251.
76. Wendy Dasler Johnson, "Cultural Rhetorics of Women's Corsets," *Rhetoric Review* 20, no. 3/4 (Autumn 2001): 203–233.
77. Cited in Kimberly Wahl, *Dressed as in a Painting: Women and British Aestheticism in an Age of Reform* (Boston: University Press of New England 2013), 13.
78. Heather Bigg and LætitiaH Andrew-Bird. "Civilization and the Corset." *The Lancet* 174, no. 4500 (November 1909): 1630–1631.
79. Cecil Fish, "Civilization and the Corset." *The Lancet* 174, no. 4502 (December 1909): 1774–1775.
80. Heather Bigg, "Civilization and the Corset." *The Lancet* 175, no. 4507 (January 1910): 203–205.
81. H. O. Kendall and F. P. Kendall, "Developing and Maintaining Good Posture," *Physical Therapy* 48, no. 4 (April 1968): 319–336, here 320.
82. Ibid., 320.
83. See the turn to a social rather than a medical definition of disability and the meaning of posture in Tobin Siebers, *Disability Theory* (Ann Arbor: Michigan University Press, 2008), relevant material on 58. See also Lennard J. Davis, *Bending Over Backwards: Disability, Dismodernism and Other Difficult Positions*, 1st Edition. (New York: NYU Press, 2002); Sharon L. Snyder, Brenda Brueggemann, and Rosemarie Garland-Thomson, eds., *Disability Studies: Enabling the Humanities* (CITY?: Modern Language Association of America, 2002).
84. Full citation?
85. Laura Smith, Elizabeth L. Weiss, and Don Lehmkuhl, *Brunnstrom's Clinical Kinesiology*, 5th ed. (Philadelphia: F. A. Davis Company, 1996).
86. Moshé Feldenkrais, *Body and Mature Behavior; a Study of Anxiety, Sex, Gravitation & Learning* (New York: International Universities Press, 1949), here 34.
87. Anson Rabinbach, *The Human Motor: Energy, Fatigue, and the Origins of Modernity* (Berkeley: University of California Press, 1991).
88. See Robert A. Yelle, "The Rhetoric of Gesture in Cross-Cultural Perspective," *Gesture* 6 (2006): 223–40; Mary Baine Campbell, "Anthropometamorphosis: John Bulwer's Monsters of Cosmetology and the Science of Culture," in Jeffrey Jerome Cohen, ed., *Monster Theory: Reading Culture* (Minneapolis: University of Minnesota Press, 1996), 202–22.
89. Robert Burton, *The Anatomy of Melancholy: What It Is, with All the Kinds, Causes, Symptomes, Prognostickes & Severall Cures of It.* (New York: Vintage Books, 1977), here 211–212.
90. Johann Jakob Schudt, *Jüdische Merkwürdigkeiten*. Vol. 2. (Frankfurt am Main: S. T. Hocker, 1718), here 368.
91. Balduin Groller, "Die körperliche Minderwertigkeit der Juden," *Die Welt* 16 (April 19, 1901): 3–5, here 4.
92. Ibid., 4.
93. Eva Brinkschulte, Muniz de Faria, and Yara Lemke. "Patienten im Atelier: die fotografische Sammlung des Arztes Heimann Wolff Berend 1858 bis 1865," *Fotogeschichte* 80 (June 2001): 17–27.

94. Max Nordau, *Degeneration* (New York: D. Appleton, 1895), here 11.
95. Cited by Todd Samuel Presner, "'Clear Heads, Solid Stomachs, and Hard Muscles': Max Nordau and the Aesthetics of Jewish Regeneration," *Modernism/modernity* 10, no. 2 (2003): 269–296, here 296.
96. Paul R. Mendes-Flohr, Jehuda Reinharz, eds., *The Jew in the Modern World: A Documentary History* (New York: Oxford University Press, 2011), 547.
97. Max Simon Nordau and Gustav Gottheil, *Zionism and Anti-Semitism* (New York Fox, Duffield & Company, 1905), 45.
98. Op. cit., 176.
99. Alex Bein, *Theodor Herzl: Biographie.* (Wien: Selbstverl. der Österreichisch-Israelischen Gesellschaft, 1974), here 173.
100. Paul Higate, *Military Masculinities: Identity and the State.* (Westport: Praeger, 2003), here 189.
101. Sharon Gillerman, "Samson in Vienna: The Theatrics of Jewish Masculinity," *Jewish Social Studies* 9, no. 2 (2003): 65–98, here 85.
102. Elias Auerbach, "Die Militärtauglichkeit der Juden," *Jüdische Rundschau* 50 (1908), 491–92.
103. Max Zirker, "Vom Basler Schauturnen," *Die jüdische Turnzeitung* no. 9 (1903): 164–9.
104. Anatole Leroy-Beaulieu and Frances Hellman, *Israel Among the Nations : a Study of the Jews and Antisemitism* (New York: G. P. Putnam's Sons; London: W. Heinemann, 1895), here 198).
105. Joseph Pennell, "The Jew at Home," *Illustrated London News* (19 December 1891): 807.
106. The translation is by Jack Zipes, Oskar Panizza, "The Operated Jew," *New German Critique* 21 (1980): 63–79, here 64.
107. M. Kohn, *The Race Gallery: The Return of Racial Science* (London: Jonathan Cape, 1995), here 36.
108. Peter Longreich, *Heinrich Himmler: A Life* (Oxford: Oxford University Press, 2013), here 600–601.
109. Keith A. Livers, *Constructing The Stalinist Body: Fictional Representations of Corporeality In The Stalinist 1930s* (Lanham, MD: Lexington Books: 2004), here 204.
110. George L. Mosse, *Nationalism and Sexuality: Respectability and Abnormal Sexuality in Modern Europe* (New York: H. Fertig, 1985).
111. Jan Robert Bloch, "How Can We Understand the Bends in the Upright Gait?" Capers Rubin, trans., *New German Critique* 45 (1988).
112. Rainer Traub, Harald Wiesner, and Otto Klemperer, *Gespräche mit Ernst Bloch* (Frankfurt am Main: Suhrkamp, 1975), here 123ff.
113. Susan Brownell, *Training the Body for China: Sports in the Moral Order of the People's Republic* (Chicago: University Of Chicago Press, 1995), here 10.
114. Karl Friedrich A. Gützlaff, *A Sketch of Chinese History, Ancient and Modern: Comprising a Retrospect of the Foreign Intercourse and Trade with China* (London: Smith, Elder and Co., 1834), here 54.
115. William Hamilton Jefferys and James L. Maxwell, *The Diseases of China: including Formosa and Korea*, (Philadelphia: P. Blakiston's Son & Company, 1911), 305–6.
116. Jing Tsu, *Failure, Nationalism, and Literature: The Making of Modern Chinese Identity, 1895–1937* (Redwood City, CA: Stanford University Press, 2005).

117. Lu Xun quoted in James Reeve Pusey, *China and Charles Darwin*, (Cambridge: Harvard University Asia Center, 1983), here 16.
118. L. A. Rocha, "Sex, Eugenics, Aesthetics, Utopia in the Life and Work of Zhang Jingsheng (1888–1970)," (Ph.D. Diss., University of Cambridge, 2010).
119. Madalina Yuk-Ling Lee, "The Intellectual Origins of Lin Yutang's Cultural Internationalism, 1928–1938," PhD Diss. University of Maryland, 2009, 116–118.
120. See Benjamin I. Schwartz, *In Search of Wealth and Power: Yen Fu and the West* (Cambridge: Belknap Press of Harvard University Press, 1964) and James Reeve Pusey, *China and Charles Darwin* (Cambridge: Harvard University Asia Center, 1983).
121. Chen Duxiu. "Jinride Jiaoyo Fanghen" (1915). In The Objectives of a Modern Education), *New Youth (Xin Qingnian)* 1 (Tokyo Daian reprint, 1962): 118.
122. Frank Dikotter, *Sex, Culture and Modernity in China: Medical Science and the Construction of Sexual Identities in the Early Republican Period.* (Honolulu: University of Hawaii Press, 1995), here 175.
123. A complete French translation of Mao's essay, along with explanatory notes and an introduction, was published by Stuart Schram, *Mao Zedong: Une Etude de l'Education Physique* (Paris/The Hague: Mouton, 1962).
124. Selected Works of Mao Tse-tung: "A Study of Physical Education." ("Tiyu zhi yonjiu"). http://www. marxists.org/reference/archive/mao/selected-works/volume-6/mswv6_01.htm. Accessed November 8, 2013.
125. Mao Tse-tung
126. Mao Tse-tung
127. Mao Tse-tung
128. Amos Elon, *Herzl* (New York: Holt, Rinehart and Winston, 1975), 63.
129. Konrad Hugo Jarausch, *Students, Society, and Politics in Imperial Germany: The Rise of Academic Illiberalism* (Princeton, NJ: Princeton University Press, 1982), here 350.
130. Ibid., 272.
131. Mao Tse-tung
132. See Zhou Xun, *Chinese Perceptions of the Jews' and Judaism: A History of the Youtai* (New York: Routledge, 2000).
133. Anonymous, "Foot-Binding," *Medical News* 41 (22 Aug 1882), 242–3, here 242.
134. Andrew D. Morris, *Marrow of the Nation: A History of Sport and Physical Culture in Republican China* (Berkeley: University of California Press, 2004).
135. P. Reginald Hug, "Posture Queen Contests in Alabama," *Journal of Chiropractic Humanities* 15 (2008): 67–80, here 72.
136. John F. Kasson, *Rudeness and Civility: Manners in Nineteenth-Century Urban America* (New York: Hill and Wang, 1991).
137. Donna J. Haraway, *Modest_Witness@Second_Millennium. FemaleMan_Meets_OncoMouse: Feminism and Technoscience* (New York: Routledge, 1997), here 142.
138. Judith Butler, *Bodies That Matter: On the Discursive Limits of "Sex."* (City: Psychology Press, 1993), here ix.

Questions

Define posture.

Who defines a good posture?

How does posture define health?

How does posture define beauty?

How does posture define the good citizen?

Can you remake someone into a good citizen by reshaping his or her posture?

Does posture mean something different in nineteenth- and early-twentieth-century China than in Western Europe?

Case Four

Obesity across Cultures

Problems: In a world in which, according to public health authorities and the media, everyone seems to be getting fatter, what does fat mean when we look across cultures? Is being fat the same in China as in the United States? How does obesity map onto culture in a world in which there are multiple, competing models for understanding illness?

Epidemics and "Imperial" Science Today

Scientists at the annual meeting of the American Association for the Advancement of Science in February 2002 warned the American government that obesity had become a "global epidemic"—no longer confined to Western, industrialized societies.[1] This warning reflected a growing consensus in the 1990s that obesity (not smoking) was going to be the major public health issue of the new millennium.[2] By 2005 the "war against obesity" had replaced the "war against tobacco," even though worldwide tobacco sales continued to increase. While obesity's status as a mass phenomenon was cemented at of the end of the last century, the phrase "war against obesity, sloth, and addiction" appeared in the UK in the broadly read, conservative newspaper *The Times* as early as 1981.[3] By the twenty-first century it was this war against obesity that had come to be seen as an epidemic by public health authorities in the West.

The People's Republic of China today has also come to see obesity as its primary health concern. But does "epidemic obesity" have the same nuances in China as it does in the West? The "obesity epidemic" seems to be the next great fear of Chinese public health officers, eclipsed only by smoking. According to recent surveys, "an obesity epidemic is imminent, with more than 20% of children aged 7–17 years in big cities now overweight or obese."[4] While the official Chinese journal of preventive medicine, *Zhonghua yufang yixue zazhi*, acknowledged that the prevalence and increment of this problem varied from rural to urban areas, it estimated that "70 million overweight and 30 million obese Chinese people emerged in China from 1992 to 2002" and that the number affected had increased rapidly in the past decade, to 260 million Chinese people, and would continue to increase without effective intervention.[5]

The shift seems to be marked. According to the Chinese public health literature, a body-mass index of greater than 25 kg/m^2 is found in 18.7 percent of the population in urban areas as opposed to 13.7 percent in rural areas. (We should note that a BMI of 30 is conventionally held to be obese.) It is not only the current state of affairs that is striking, but the rapid increase in obesity seen over the past decades. These figures are for 1997. They mark a fourfold increase over 1982 when only 3.7 percent of Chinese adults had a BMI of over 25.[6] Chinese medical and epidemiological studies argue that "obesity has become a global epidemic," though there seems to be little knowledge of the state of affairs in China (meaning the People's Republic of China). Looking at "a group of 2776 randomly selected adults (20–94 years of age) living in the Huayang Community in Shanghai, China," a 2002 study argued that while "the prevalence of obesity [using Western standards] was lower in China than in the West, "overall fat mass-related metabolic disorders were also common."[7] The Chinese data seemed to show the disease patterns traditionally associated with obesity in the West, such as an increase in type 2 diabetes, seemed somewhat independent of the rate of obesity in China.

Obesity is *the* problem of the twenty-first century, but is it truly a "Chinese" problem, or is obesity—which is clearly seen as *a* problem in China—a Western problem read through a Chinese lens? Is this apparent epidemic in China merely the importation of a Western model of health and illness or a reconfiguration in Chinese terms? This chapter examines the epidemic of obesity in China in relation to the historical background provided by nineteenth- and twentieth-century engagements between China and the West. Though never entirely colonized by Western powers and Japan, much of mainland China was, in the early twentieth century, part of Europe's "informal empire," and relations with these intruding nation-states were marked by the stark power imbalance that was a characteristic of formal colonial rule elsewhere. Allopathic medicine was one of the major tools from the beginning of the nineteenth century for the establishment of a Western cultural hegemony in China. This chapter addresses the question of how the circulation of Western medical and health discourses helped shape Chinese self-awareness during the period leading to the present acceptance of discourses of public health in the PRC. It builds upon recent studies foregrounding the importance of Western medicine to the formation of Chinese ideas about the body, the self, and the nation-state. In particular, it considers how constructions of obesity drew upon medical discourses circulating in modern China and were informed by cultural anxieties surrounding the import of Western commodities associated with the public's health, such as tinned milk, into China.

The "Fat" Body in China

On the surface, the fear of an epidemic of obesity seems to be a contemporary Western importation. Concern in China's immediate past as well as in the nineteenth century had centered not upon an epidemic of obesity but rather recurring epidemics of famine. James L. Watson notes that the dominant sense of fear concerning the body in modern China is the result of the experience of the great famine under Mao Zedong.[8] This famine, which lasted from 1958 to 1961 and resulted from the collectivization of peasants, killed millions in China and evoked the horrors of famines from Imperial China to the famines of the 1940s during the war against the Japanese. For adults in today's China, "famine" recalls their own experiences under Mao and the tales of starvation during the war handed down by their parents and grandparents. Mao's great famine, too, had its echoes of the famine culture attributed to and experienced in China in the nineteenth century. In such circumstances, how did obesity come to be understood?

In early-twentieth-century China there was a medical obsession with the epidemic of famine as the "famine" that had marked Western views of the pathological body in nineteenth-century China. When the standard "Western" medical journal published in China, the *China Medical Journal*, is read systematically from the beginning of the twentieth century to the Japanese invasion of China in 1937, the central medical discourse concerning "diet" and the body is that of famine and starvation. In such texts, China is truly the "sick man of Asia," as Larissa N. Heinrich discusses in her book *The Afterlife of Images: Translating the Pathological Body between*

China and the West.[9] Heinrich's book is actually an answer in part to Shigehisa Kuriyama's central thesis in his *The Expressiveness of the Body and the Divergence of Greek and Chinese Medicine* (1999) that argued for an inherent antithesis between "Western" (Greek) and "Eastern" (Chinese) images of the body and therefore between the very nature of the body in each cultural milieu. Heinrich illustrates how the rhetorical commonplace of "China as the sick man of Asia" is historically structured through the tension between Chinese high culture (including medicine) and Western claims of the inherent inferiority of that culture and Western superiority in all media of expression and representation. It is the rereading of a "sick" China through Western medicine and its illustrations that preoccupies Heinrich and as such she provides an important corrective to Kuriyama's view.

For Kuriyama, the "model" body type in classical Chinese medical literature and culture is described as rotund, in opposition to the muscular and svelte bodies of Greek art and medicine. Heinrich shows how Western models of the "sick" Chinese body came to be accepted within China as an adequate representation of the very nature of what it meant to be Chinese despite (according to Heinrich) evidence to the contrary. The difference between Kuriyama and Heinrich, of course, lies in the historical periods examined by both—Kuriyama examines the ancient roots of both the West and the East, in contexts where contact between the two was extremely limited; Heinrich's book examines the post-Enlightenment world, the height of massive colonial expansion into Asia. The "sick man of Asia" is the result of experiences of famine and malnourishment in a world reshaped by colonial expansion.

Thus when we look at famine in China it takes on two quite different meanings as an epidemic: for the classical world of Chinese medicine it is caused by an imbalance in nature and in the body; for the modern world it is—as indicated by the food tickets circulated by the Chinese Communist Party in Shanghai in 1927 stating that the British were responsible for the famine—the result of colonial oppression and its impact on the world of food. In nineteenth and early-twentieth-century China, epidemic and famine were widely seen as interlinked no mater how both were defined.[10]

Western medicine in the new age of bacteriology of the late nineteenth century, of Koch and Pasteur, also sees widespread famine and infectious epidemics as linked. According to William Hamilton Jefferys and James L. Maxwell:

> in the summer of 1906 there was a frightfully fatal and widespread epidemic of subtertian malaria all over Hupeh and Hunan, owing, it is believed, to a famine in Honan the previous winter which drove southward a hundred thousand or more starving Honanese, whose depressed vitality it is supposed afforded the fertile soil necessary to light up the epidemic. At least this is the theory held by those who report from these provinces.[11]

Here we see not famine as an epidemic but famine as tied to models of epidemic.

Famine and Cure

In nineteenth- and early-twentieth-century China the physicians of the Chinese Medical Missionary Association were concerned with the outcome of such epidemics. They needed to develop models for the treatment of the sequelae of famine, and they turned, not surprisingly, to those advocated by allopathic medicine. They were concerned with ensuring that the food made available in their hospitals had sufficient protein and fat, to the extent that they advocated tactics such as "crossing foreign and native cows" or introducing canned milk to improve the local diet.[12] Modern treatment being advocated for contending with an ancient and endemic problem. Canned, condensed milk, as the historian of twentieth-century China Frank Dikötter notes, was "modern" in China in the nineteenth century and became a sign of the adaptation of China to the modern world.[13] But it was also a sign of an early attempt to remedy a Chinese "problem" with a Western solution. Condensed milk presented what was considered by some to be the perfect food in the light of the claims of nineteenth century science that cows' milk had a therapeutic influence upon a range of illnesses.[14] In this way, the American neurologist S. Weir Mitchell noted in his 1877 *Fat and Blood*: "Milk is the best and most easily managed addition to a general diet."[15] Certainly in 1877, raw milk, unpasteurized and a source of infectious diseases, was anything but a real health food. (While Louis Pasteur and Claude Bernard developed pasteurization for wine in 1864, its broad use for milk was not introduced until much later. Indeed, Robert Koch saw pasteurization of cow's milk as unnecessary, as he believed well into the twentieth century that bovine tuberculosis could not be transmitted by milk to human beings.)

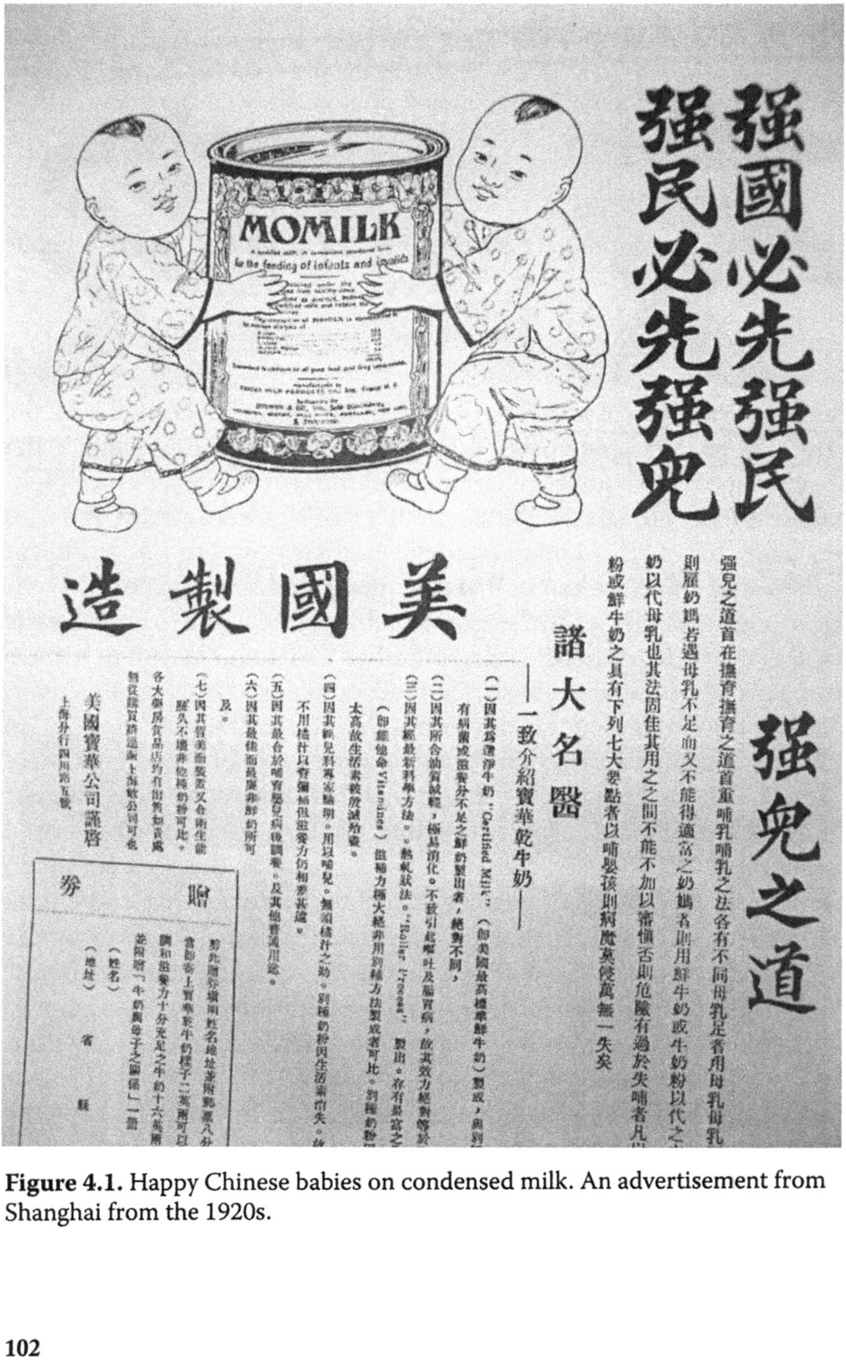

Figure 4.1. Happy Chinese babies on condensed milk. An advertisement from Shanghai from the 1920s.

Condensed milk is, however, a very poor substitute for mother's milk, given the extremely high percentage of sugar found in it. "Preserved condensed milk is simply a combination of sugar and condensed milk, in which the value of the sugar is greater than the value of the condensed milk," noted John G. Borden, the son of its inventor Gail Borden, in 1885.[16] Condensed milk, like boiled water, was not only concentrated but was inadvertently pasteurized (as the process for condensing milk was developed in 1856 well before Pasteur) and was therefore perceived as a healthy alternative food. Yet cow's milk was not the "perfect food" for the treatment of famine-related diseases in China. Given the "frequency of decreased lactase activity ranges [of] 95% for Han Chinese,"[17] one would imagine that canned milk might actually have had deleterious effects for those infants with greater lactose intolerance so fed.

Why was a substitute for mother's milk sought in this world of epidemic famine? Were physicians dealing with the epidemic of famine concerned only with the failure of infants to thrive? According to William Hamilton Jefferys and James L. Maxwell in 1911:

> The Chinese child is devotedly cared for, but after that period of absolute dependence its parental attentions undergo marked deterioration and it does a lot of shifting for itself. One gets the impression that most Chinese babies are born with excellent health and are particularly round and fat and chubby; and though congenital deformities are not uncommonly met with, congenital disease is comparatively rarely so.[18]

For:

> the Chinese mother knows nothing of modified milk mixtures and artificial feeding rarely, if ever, crosses the horizon of her thought. In the case of the well-to-do if the mother's milk is insufficient, she readily acquires the cooperation of a wet nurse. In the case of the poor, there is the aunt or the sister-in-law living in the same house with a baby or two of her own, ready to supply the deficiency. We have not infrequently seen the grandmother turned to in such straits—possibly the great grandmother occasionally takes a turn![19]

And thus condensed milk emerged as the answer. Plump babies were understood as healthy babies. Yet concerns remained that the seeming health of the Chinese infant might merely be a sham, quickly giving way to further diseases.

Debates about famine reflect often on the "peculiarities" of the Chinese. Sometimes the differences were seen in terms of geography and class: the Chinese diet was regionally differentiated and appeared to compensate for levels of wealth. One physician noted that the "rich have rice, vegetables, and meats. The poor have rice, vegetables and substitutes for meat." It was only "when floods overtake the people year in and year out that so many are driven to our doors for charity."[20] China was from this perspective not a "famine" culture at all. Rather, from the standpoint of the physicians, it was the distribution of food by the Chinese, especially in times of turmoil or disaster, that seemed to lie at the heart of episodes of famine. In this view, the failure of the local Chinese distribution network is the cause of famine.[21] The suspicion remained among Western physicians in China that indigenous foods might not be "suitable" enough to maintain a healthy diet.[22] The soybean was advocated over and over again as a substitute for other forms of protein, as if by virtue of repetition Western physicians might be convinced of its virtues/suitability.[23]

Yet when the concern was true starvation the sense that "Western" cures, such as a rich, milk-based diet were most appropriate reappeared among members of the medical community.[24] Children were seen as most at risk from the effects of famine, both in terms of the deleterious effects of hunger and the pernicious actions of its intransigent parents. The selling of children was closely connected with, and seen as a major consequence of, the famine culture in China.[25] "Cannot the famine relief associations . . . take this matter into consideration and put an end to it," wrote one irate physician in 1920.[26] Among the myriad concerns expressed about the pathological effects of diet, not a single word was spent on the dangers or effects of our modern concern about the epidemic of obesity.[27]

Western Views of Obesity in the Land of Famine

Yet, from the mid-nineteenth century China, the "sick man of Asia," was imagined by Westerners as inhabiting a land of obesity and the Chinese as an obese people. In 1849, Jean-Pierre Beaude stated that the Chinese hold "a man . . . in dignity regards embonpoint and even obesity as one of the requirements of his rank." This was because obesity was believed to be the result of a wealthy and pampered status, bringing with it access to an excess and variety of foodstuffs.[28] The Chinese, it was claimed, held a belief that the prosperous and powerful man must be "one who really fills up a chair."[29] From the mid-nineteenth century, however, obesity began to be reread as a symptom of decadence and degeneracy. Frederic W. Farrar stated that obesity was a mark of Chinese developmental inferiority: "The unmarked features, the serene, blandly-smiling face, the tendency to physical obesity and mental apathy, the feeble, tranquil, childish, gluttonous sensuality, mark the race."[30] Unlike the healthy and hardy European, Arthur de Gobineau claimed, the Chinese were fat and indolent, the people most often likely to be obese.[31]

Chinese obesity thus emerged as a marker of the quality of race as well as a social practice. According to one Western source:

> In China there is every variety of climate, food and social condition.... The whole race displays a remarkable tendency to obesity. The nutritious juices of the body are directed towards the surface, distending and overloading the cellular tissues with inordinate quantity of fat. This general tendency of the whole people can only be attributed to the hereditary diathesis, unchecked by intermarriage with others differently constituted. It is an evil which exclusiveness of that singular people has entailed upon them.[32]

According to J. Richardson Parke, the Chinese were fascinated with obesity as part of their ideals of sexuality:

> In almost all Oriental countries the "stout lady" is in demand. In fact there are portions of our own where the supply sometimes runs short; but in Turkey and China, where the highest social and matrimonial ambitions are not realized so much through the spirituelle type of feminine loveliness as by the number of fingers of fat over the ribs, the ladies are shut up and stall-fed, like Strasbourg geese, before their prudent parents think of putting them upon the market. Indeed the pashas and mandarins, who are the chief patrons of this nourishing domestic industry, buying their wives in carload lots, and always on trial, are not as a rule highly spirituelle themselves, running to stomach rather than soul, and paying far greater heed to quantity than to quality.[33]

If marriage traditions were not to blame, then corrupt governance was. For Jeffreys and Maxwell: "Apoplexy among the aged officials in Peking, properly disposed to it by their obesity and their having to perform the nine obeisances before the emperor so frequently, is not very uncommon."[34] While they were obese, unlike the Jews ("a diabetic people") who have also been represented as suffering from diseases of excess because of their race and marriage practices, the Chinese were less often seen to suffer from diseases attendant to obesity, such as diabetes. Hence, for Thomas B. Futcher:

> All authorities agree that the Hebrew race is particularly susceptible. Frerichs states that of his 400 cases 102 were Jews. Wallach clearly demonstrated its greater frequency among the Hebrews of Frankfurt. From 1872 to 1890 there were 171 deaths from diabetes in that city. The proportion 674 of deaths from diabetes to the deaths from all causes was six times greater among the Jews than among the rest of the inhabitants. The factors occasioning this greater susceptibility in Hebrews are not well understood. It has been variously ascribed to greater instability of the nervous system, fondness for sweets, and overeating and sedentary habits particularly among the better classes. Diabetes is very common among the educated and commercial classes in India, and Rose and Sen have shown that it is the Hindoos who chiefly suffer. The disease is said to be very uncommon in China and Japan.[35]

This is somewhat odd given that the Chinese diet was seen as encouraging such pathological developments. Fuchter added:

> We might suppose that the prolonged excessive use of carbohydrate food would favor the development of diabetes. There seems no satisfactory evidence favoring this view, however. Cantani stated that the majority of his Italian patients subsisted largely on farinaceous food. He believed the diet was an important etiological factor. In Ceylon, also, where diabetes is common, large quantities of saccharine food are taken. The Chinese, on the other hand, rarely suffer from diabetes, although their diet consists chiefly of carbohydrates.[36]

In the argument over whether "fat" or "carbohydrates" were most at fault for obesity and the diseases attendant to obesity, carbohydrates were more often blamed following the great popular success of William Banting's dieting practices at midcentury that advocated a radical reduction in the consumption of what he called *farinaceous* foods.

This obsession of Western medical professionals based in China with the obesity of the Chinese reappears in the popular Chinese press of the late Qing and the Republican period as China becomes "modern."

Though the concern with obesity also appeared in Chinese-language periodicals wherein it may be seen as a response to the past and contemporary, allopathic medicine view of China as a famine culture, it did so in the form of articles by foreigners freely adapted and purveyed for consumption in these journals and magazines. While a minority voice in the world of Western allopathic medicine viewing China, the concern with the fat Chinese body was consistently voiced as a sign of the inherent disparities of indigenous society.

Obesity in China: Traditional and Revolutionary Views

Obesity seems not to have been a major problem in the various theories of the ill body in Chinese medicine. There was, however, a constant and intense concern with the "immoderate body" in the medical and dietetic literature of traditional Chinese medicine. In the sixteenth century Li Shizhen (1518–1593) wrote in his *Bencai gangmu* (Systematic Materia Medica) that the consumption of fresh crabs was healthy "in small quantities" but:

> Gluttons will consume a dozen or more at a sitting together with various kinds of meat and other foods. They eat and drink twice as much as they need . . . then blame [their upset stomachs on] the crabs. But why blame the crabs?[37]

The culture of excess in the world of traditional Chinese medicine became a hallmark of the degenerate Chinese body in need of regeneration by the early twentieth century. This was quite in contrast to the cultural anxiety about emaciation, which drove thin people to undertake "special bulking diets" in order to find marriage partners. Such emaciation was often seen as the curse of ancestors who were:

> "Eating" the health and vitality of a descendant in retaliation for neglect or mistreatment. Plumpness, by contrast, was perceived as a clear indication that the person so blessed was in harmony with the supernatural world.[38]

In the writings of Western commentators in early-twentieth-century China, the dominant image of China as a starvation culture thus had its answer in the counterexample of the degenerate obese body.

Immediately before the revolution that overthrew the Qing dynasty on October 10, 1911, "reform" was everywhere. As a new fantasy of the "reformed" body began to emerge in China, obesity came to be viewed as one of the signs of the degenerate Chinese body, a body clearly in need of reform. Following the model of "regeneration" that captured most of the ideologies of the day (from Zionism to Marxism to Social Darwinism to Colonialism), interventions concerning obesity defined the ability of the society to reform the individual. In one of the most widely read columns, "Ziyoutan" (unfettered talk), in the renowned newspaper *Shenbao*, the author Wang Dungen, a well-known writer and a key figure in the "Mandarin Ducks and Butterflies School" explored the reform of the body. In the late 1910s and early 1920s, Wang Dungen was under attack by the progressive writers of the May Fourth movement, and in 1914 he created the comic journal *Saturday* in which he responded to his critics. In a comic essay entitled, "Reforming the Human Body," Wang Dungen envisioned a grotesque ideal of the "new" body comprising a newly configured mouth, tongue, ear, eyes, nose, skin, eyebrows, hair, teeth, neck, shoulders, arms, hands, fingers, and feet. The new body possessed hundreds of mouths so that its owner could eat more and yet still be able to talk.[39] This was an ironic response to the starved body, a body desiring reform so that it might consume ever more, and it emerged at a moment when calls were being advanced for the adoption of "Western" models of regeneration, such as structured physical exercise, as a means of reforming the too-fat body. Chen Duxiu, the leader of the New Cultural Movement, advocated exercise to make the Chinese physically as well as morally fit, and Mao Zedong in 1917 published a full-scale essay on physical education as a means to reform the body.[40]

By 1913, the classical Chinese medical literature on obesity was beginning to be summarized for an intellectual readership in China. The essay "On Obesity," by Shu Hui and Wei Seng, written in classical Chinese, was published in a leading women's magazine. Such magazines shaped and were shaped by the images of the so-called "New Woman" (*xin nuxing*) and "Westernized Modern Girl" (*modeng nulang*) that came into prominence in the first decade of the twentieth century in China as well as in the West. These images were defined in many ways, but to no little extent by their "thin" body form. Thinness, even after the establishment of the People's Republic, as James L. Watson has noted, continued to be a mark of "bad luck, illness, and early death."[41] Thinness was the "stigma of emaciation" that scarred the psyche of the Chinese at the beginning and the close of the twentieth century. The thin body was associated not with "modern" thought, but with village superstition and backwardness among the intellectuals of the early twentieth-century.

The "On Obesity" essay of 1913 presented the argument that obesity was an illness that women should not take lightly.[42] The authors referred to figures from ancient China, including a man named "Zilong" who lived in the Warring States period. Considering himself to be too fat, Zilong took *Phragmites communis Trirn* (a traditional medicine) to lose weight. The authors offered this example to prove that obesity was an illness treatable by medical intervention even in the premodern period. One of their sources was *Hanshu* (*The History of the Former Han*

Dynasty), written by the historian Bangu. They argued that according to Hanshu, too much body fat is the cause of obesity. But there are two kinds of obesity; one associated with a surfeit and another of a deficit of blood cells. The causes of the former were not eating appropriately, not having a balanced lifestyle, and not having enough sex. Not eating appropriately meant that one ate too many unhealthy foods such as flour, sugar, and alcohol. Obesity of the second type was caused by external injury, overworking, or stress, and sometimes occurred after giving birth.

As with the Western medical literature of the late nineteenth century, free adaptations of articles from the Western press advanced the idea that there are stages of obesity.[43] For the authors of the 1913 essay, for example, obesity had three phases. In the initial phase, the person would look acceptably plump, which, since it was taken as a sign of prosperity, would mean that others would admire him; in the next phase, he would begin to look overtly obese and would thus take on a comical appearance; and finally, in the last phase his life would be in danger and others would take pity on him. This final stage of obesity would present with symptoms including sweating, fatigue, backache, heart disease, sexual incompetence, and so forth. The "cure" for obesity was a balanced diet and lifestyle: avoiding eating things containing too much fat, not sleeping for more than eight hours, taking a warm bath two or three times a week, walking two or three hours every day, and being persistent. The condition could be medicated with either a traditional cure, such as *wodu*, or, better yet, thyroid tablets. The latter offered the classical pharmaceutical intervention and certainly could reduce weight—by making the individual hyperthyroidal and increasing the basal metabolism. While this would lead to weight loss, it could also lead to a wide range of other pathologies, such as Graves' disease.

The treatment of obesity as an endocrinological deficiency, one of the most up-to-date views of early-twentieth-century medicine, is suggestive of the way that modern ideas were creeping into classical Chinese views on obesity. The obese body was held by Western observers to be the antithesis of the beautiful and healthy body. Therefore, it presented a special problem for contemporary women. In an essay "Keep the Body Slim," adapted and published in a women's magazine in 1922, the author, Dai Zuo, stressed that people with obesity were not beautiful, especially women: "A person who is too fat looks very ugly. Women especially can't be fat. If a woman gains too much weight and became fatty, where can one find her beauty?"[44] In addition, obesity was coming to be seen as an important medical problem. Obesity was the result of faulty metabolism, the result of a hormone imbalance. Yet obesity was not a random occurrence. Certain people were more at risk than others: specifically people who ate rich food in abundance, people who are not physically active, people with a family inheritance of obesity, and, of course, alcoholics.

The essay made clear that obesity was dangerous because it led to heart disease. People with obesity had shortness of breath and rapid heartbeats after walking even a few steps. They were more likely to have a stroke. People with obesity also had urinary and kidney problems. Dieting offered the solution. The essay advised one should not overeat, avoiding food that contained too much fat and eating less meat. Other suggestions it provided for weight loss were engaging in physical exercise and using laxatives and electric steam therapy to reduce body fat, which, according to the essay, was very popular abroad. Electrotherapy certainly was a standard late-nineteenth-century Western treatment for the "failure or perversion of nutrition," including diabetes.[45]

Women were the clear targets of the growing anti-obesity anxiety of Republican China. Chinese intellectuals, as with intellectuals and politicians in Western national states in this period, were focused on what was perceived as a decline in birth rate among the elites. Women's bodies were the focus of a range of concerns, from the impact of intellectual life on reproduction to the growing sense that obese elites could not reproduce healthy children. In one essay the author, Zhou Zhenyu, stated that he was a doctor who often had female patients who needed help to lose weight. Zhou Zhenyu commented, "when I was a doctor in Beiping [the older spelling of Beijing], I often had women patients come asking for the method of losing weight. I would tell them the method, some of them went home and practiced following my suggestions, others would come visit again and want medication. The effects differ because the causes of their obesity vary."[46] "The cause and danger of female obesity" (as Zhou Zhenyu labeled it) was seen either in terms of overindulgence and the absence of exercise or an imbalance of the hormones.

This is the classic argument about obesity that dominated the late-nineteenth-century discussion of its causes. In the United States, the home of most of the medical missionaries based in China, the editors of the *Journal of the American Medical Association* published a 1924 editorial entitled "What Causes Obesity?" In it they argued, following a powerful anti-psychological strand in obesity research that began in the late nineteenth century, for an etiology of obesity rooted in malfunctions of normal metabolic processes. See obesity as a "scientific problem," they wrote, and that will free the "fat woman" from the stigma for which she "has the remedy in her own hands—or rather between her own teeth." That new object of scientific interest was the fat woman, who had been charged with carrying "that extra weight about with her unless she so wills."[47] Women, not "men" or "people" were considered to be most at risk from obesity, a far cry from the evocation of Falstaff as the exemplary sufferer from obesity in the mid-nineteenth century. According to an article published in the *Journal of the American Medical Association* in 1922, although fat people usually ate less than thin people, they did not burn enough calories. Large amounts of fat were accumulated and stored in their bodies. While the obese did not eat much at every meal, they often ate between meals. Women specifically could suffer from hypothyroidism, hypopituitarism, or a loss of estrogen. Pregnant women were especially at risk. One woman, after giving birth, had to get up and eat every night. She quickly gained weight and became obese.

The danger of female obesity is the collapse of one's health and thus one's ability to bear children. This remains the classic definition of women's health. Obese women have compromised immune systems and are likely to catch colds and coughs, which leads to tuberculosis. They have heart disease. Their nervous systems are endangered. The obese are usually slow and lazy, but often they laugh and appear jovial. A disease that can be triggered by pregnancy ends up preventing conception, causing sexual problems, and heightening the possibility of miscarriage.

By 1941, as war raged and famine haunted China, a public discourse on obesity articulated by Western medical professionals was woven into the new "reformed" Chinese attitude toward the body. These attitudes came to be labeled as a "tragedy at the dinner table."[48] It is always difficult to judge how widespread such views were among the urban elites, but the indication that such concerns were read in the popular press may be seen as an indication of the acceptance of such ideas about the fat body, at least among this readership. An essay, another free adaptation among a number of foreign medical and popular articles, especially those authored by American experts, appeared in the Chinese popular review, *Liangyou*, bearing this title. It presented the pathological consequences of overeating. The author identified middle-aged people as being most at risk, because they seemed to be more easily attracted to fine dining. The essay defined pathology by quoting a saying attributed to an American congressman: "fifty, fifty, fifty," which means if a fifty-year-old person is fifty pounds overweight, his life span will be reduced by 50 percent. The author also quoted statistics provided by an American doctor suggesting that out of two thousand cases of sudden death, 90 percent of those involved had died of heart disease. The author observed "most of them eat too much, are overweight, which causes heart disease." While other foreign cases of overeating were mentioned in the article, such as the ancient Romans, the American Thanksgiving was given special mention as a moment of extreme public gluttony:

> Around Thanksgiving time, there are often cases of death caused by overeating to be found in the mortuary. People in charge of the postmortem examinations are often too busy rushing to luxurious banquets to do their work. It's also quite dangerous to eat too much after fasting. One should definitely divide all the nice dishes into several meals, and never eat everything at once. It is nice to be able to enjoy a full table of luxurious food, but one should remember not to gamble with one's own life. Otherwise tragedy would take place in the holiday season, and one would sadly fall onto the bosom of the death.

The result of such gluttony was sudden death, chronic heart disease, or diabetes. A litany of diseases was said to be the result of obesity: high blood pressure, lung disease, cancer, even suicide and accidental death. For, according to the author, people with obesity often had psychological problems and were very slow in reacting to what was going on around them—and thus were prone to accidents. The overweight individual was advised to consult qualified doctors to monitor his or her individual diet. Yet the "cure" proposed in the essay of 1941 was to pay minute attention to what and how much one ate. The formula did not have much to do with any specific type of food, rather the idea that as one grew older, one should eat less. By the time one was very old, one should only eat light and simple food, returning in effect to the kind of diet prescribed for infants.

China, like America, seems to be suffering from a new epidemic of obesity but one that now documents its modernity—no model of Oriental, primitive infectious diseases is evident here. Rather there is a claim of the "invasion from the West." Earlier negative depictions of obesity as a reflection of inherent Chinese problems—whether social or racial as seen through the eyes of Western observers and consumed by readers of Chinese magazines—becomes a model for this undesirable circulation. The consumption of modern Western products such as condensed milk, seen initially as a potential cure for the diseases resulting from famine, come to be read as the cause of this new urban and Western phenomenon of obesity. However, the negative aspects of the new economy imported from the West could be addressed and confronted through the importation of models of obesity derived from Western public health. Obesity and its treatment could thus be understood as part of a system of modernization wherein all of the pitfalls of modern living were apparent, and the cure apparent and available for consumption. Like concepts such as famine, obesity, too, was rooted in China in nineteenth- and early-twentieth-century understandings of health and illness. Evoking the "Western" causes of obesity, Chinese public health officials today echo this older, Chinese model of an obesity epidemic—for all that is bad in Chinese health must still have its roots in the West.

Implications of the Transnational Obesity Discussion

There are practical policy issues that are reflected in the problems in the continuities and ruptures of the image of the obese and obesity.[49] In contemporary China obesity has become a general public health concern, with more than 20 percent youth obesity reported in urban areas.[50] Indeed there seems to be a consensus that rapid changes in body mass have occurred over the past few decades, and this has had major, deleterious health effects.[51] Indeed between 1989 and 2000, obesity rates doubled among women in China and tripled among men.[52] Indeed the argument that cultural attitudes toward overweight and single children in China—specifically, the association of fatness with prosperity and health and the "one child policy"—that may make being overweight socially acceptable is acknowledged without specific changes in policy being proposed.[53] Indeed, the privileging of male children over female children may account for higher rates of urban male child obesity in today's China.[54] Men and boys are at greater risk in China for the diseases attendant to obesity, such as type 2 diabetes. Policy considerations have focused on critiquing the importation of Western eating patterns rather than actually limiting access to such food. Even the proposed changes in the urban one-child policy endorsed by the Communist Party Central Committee in late 2013 is based on the parents being only children, not on questions of health.[55] Obesity remains seen as a problem, but one not having Chinese origins.

Such considerations seem to play little role in the debates about health care in the United States and the new health care law [HR 4872]. Assuming that the law remains basically the same as it comes into effect between now and 2015–16, one of the real questions raised will deal with whether the changes introduced will radically reduce costs and thus enable more people to get better health care. The calculus was—and this is classic Adam Smith economics—the more people you have in a pool, the fewer percentage-wise are going to get ill at any given time, and therefore the general costs will go down. Meaning, if you have healthy eighteen-year-olds in the pool, their contributions will help pay for older people with greater health problems.

Yet it is the image of the "healthy eighteen-year-old" and the "infirm elderly" that shapes such as argument. If the claims about increased obesity in children and teenagers are anywhere near accurate—I think they are more accurate than not—then we are going to experience an enormous number of younger people who will have major illnesses early on, as well as the sequelae from those illnesses. If you become diabetic when you are forty, you will have cardiovascular problems when you are sixty. If you become diabetic when you are ten that means you may already be ill as an eighteen-year-old and later become a sick and very expensive thirty-year-old.

The disjuncture between idealized images of "normal and healthy man/woman" (an odd version of what some economists call "rational man" and the law has called "reasonable man") that haunt such reckoning can be seen in today's politics of obesity. Childhood obesity has been taken up by Michelle Obama as one of her primary interests as first lady. In her opening salvo on February 9, 2010 she commented:

> It wasn't that long ago that I was a working Mom, struggling to balance meetings and deadlines with soccer and ballet. And there were some nights when everyone was tired and hungry, and we just went to the drive-thru because it was quick and cheap, or went with one of the less healthy microwave options, because it was easy.
>
> . . . [I]t's time for a moment of truth for our country; it's time we all had a wakeup call. It's time for us to be honest with ourselves about how we got here. Our kids didn't do this to themselves. Our kids don't decide what's served to them at school or whether there's time for gym class or recess. Our kids don't choose to make food products with tons of sugar and sodium in super-sized portions, and then to have those products marketed to them everywhere they turn. And no matter how much they beg for pizza, fries and candy, ultimately, they are not, and should not, be the ones calling the shots at dinnertime. We're in charge. We make these decisions.[56]

Her view is that obesity is not a medical problem, even though it has health consequences, rather it is a social or even a moral problem (laziness). Obesity is the result of an adult lack of desire to exercise and eat well. Such views stereotype all people who are obese as lazy and stupid and unable to deal with problems that they themselves have some control over. But obesity has become a public health issue that has an ever-growing pot of money associated with it. Everybody is jockeying to get a part of that pie: the geneticists are making claims that it's all a question of genetic inheritance; the endocrinologists are arguing that this is mainly a problem of metabolic change; the infectious disease specialists point to increased obesity in those infected with specific viruses; the people interested in social medicine say if people only had better access to organic or slow food there would not be any problem with obesity—all of which, in bits and pieces, is true. The moralizers argue that we should reintroduce physical labor—now in the form of compulsory exercise regimes in schools or a "fat tax" on unhealthy food. If the first lady is heard, then obesity will be viewed as primarily a medical problem rather than a social one. Yet for some overweight people obesity is primarily a medical problem. They are not going to be helped by having access to better food and a better lifestyle. It is the image of the obese with all its history that frames these questions. Without an awareness of this history, the debates and the solutions will always be partial, fragmentary, or contradictory. Indeed, recent experimental data has shown that the public expression of the stigma of obesity can be one of its causes.

> Some policies and campaigns designed to combat obesity portray overweight and obese individuals negatively. For example, Georgia's "Strong4Life" campaign to combat childhood obesity prominently features advertisements portraying fat children as unhappy; other states send heavy children home with "BMI report cards"; and the Boy Scouts of America recently placed BMI restrictions for boys participating in the Boy Scout Jamboree. Although it may not be their primary intent, such programs increase stigmatization of overweight individuals.[57]

As a historian I am great believer that what medicine does best is to think about multiple causes for complex outcomes. And much of what I have heard over the last couple of years in the medical sciences and also in the political realm is exactly the opposite. It is simple answers and simple proposals based on an incomplete command of the vocabulary of images employed in Asia as well as in North America. This is a typical policy problem that the study of images of health and illness may help address.

Notes

1. http://www.newswise.eom/articles/2002/2/OBESITY.URI.html. (accessed 1 March 2008).
2. Ali H. Mokdad, Mary K. Serdula, William H. Dietz, Barbara A. Bowman, James S. Marks, and Jeffrey P. Koplan, "The Spread Of The Obesity Epidemic In The United States, 1991–1998," *Journal of the American Medical Association* 282 (1999): 1519–22.
3. Annabel Ferriman, "The Man Who Will Try To Persuade Us To Give Up Some Of Life's Good Things," *The Times* [London], (Friday, August 7, 1981), 12.
4. Longde Wang, Lingzhi Kong, Fan Wu, Yamin Bai and Robert Burton, "Preventing Chronic Diseases in China," *The Lancet* 366, no. 9499 (19 November 2005–25 November 2005): 1821–1824, here 1821; see also Dongfeng Gu, Kristi Reynolds, Xigui Wu, Jing Chen, Xiufang Duan, Robert F Reynolds, Paul K Whelton, Jiang He, "Prevalence of the Metabolic Syndrome and Overweight Among Adults In China" *The Lancet*, 365, no. 9468 (16 April 2005–22 April 2005): 1398–1405.
5. G. S. Ma, Y. P. Li, Y. F. Wu, et al., "[The Prevalence of Body Overweight and Obesity and Its Changes Among Chinese People during 1992 To 2002]," *Zhonghua Yu Fang Yi Xue Za Zhi* [*Chinese Journal of Preventive Medicine*] 39 (2005): 311–5.
6. Xiaoping Weng and Benjamin Caballero, *Obesity and Its Related Diseases in China: The Impact of the Nutrition Transition in Urban and Rural Adults* (Youngstown, NY: Cambria Press, 2007), 1.
7. W. P. Jia, K. S. Xiang, L. Chen, J. X. Lu and Y. M. Wu, "Epidemiological Study on Obesity and its Comorbidities in urban Chinese older than 20 years of age in Shanghai, China," *Obesity Reviews* 3 (2002): 157–165.
8. James L. Watson, "Food as a Lens: The Past, Present, and Future of Family Life in China," in Jun Jing, ed., *Feeding China's Little Emperors: Food, Children, and Social Change* (Stanford University Press, 2000), 199–212, here, 208.
9. Larissa N. Heinrich, *The Afterlife of Images: Translating the Pathological Body between China and the West* (Durham: Duke University Press, 2008).
10. Lillian M. Li, *Fighting Famine in North China: State, Market, and Environmental Decline, 1690s-1990s* (Palo Alto, CA: Stanford University Press, 2007), 264 and Robert Marks, *Tigers, Rice, Silk, And Silt: Environment and Economy In Late Imperial South China* (Cambridge: Cambridge University Press, 1998), 148.
11. William Hamilton Jefferys and James L. Maxwell, *The Diseases of China: including Formosa and Korea* (London: Bale & Danielsson), 48.
12. "Preliminary Report of Committee on Infant and Invalid Diet," *China Medical Journal* 26 (1912): 133–44.
13. Frank Dikötter, *Exotic Commodities: Modern Objects and Everyday Life in China* (New York: Columbia University Press, 2007), 220 (sweetened milk as therapy for hospital patients); 224, (the craze for condensed milk as modern).
14. Hannah Velten, *Milk: A Global History* (London: Reaktion, 2010).
15. S. Weir Mitchell, *Fat and Blood* (New York: Lippincott, 1900), 119.
16. *Testimony taken by the subcommittee on the tariff of the Senate Committee on the Tariff United States. Congress. Senate. Committee on Finance* (Washington, DC: Government Printing Office, 1885), 835.
17. N. Kretchmer "Lactose and Lactase," *Scientific American* 227, no. 4 (1972): 71–8.

18. William Hamilton Jefferys and James L. Maxwell, *The Diseases of China: including Formosa and Korea* (London: Bale & Danielsson, 1911), 259.
19. Jefferys and Maxwell, 259.
20. Mary Stone, "Hospital Dietary in China," *China Medical Journal* 26 (1912): 298–301, here 299.
21. Amartya Sen argued that famine occurs not from a lack of food, but from inequalities built into mechanisms for distributing food. Amartya Sen, *Poverty and Famines: An Essay on Entitlement and Deprivation* (Clarendon Press/Oxford University Press, Oxford, UK, 1981); B. E. Read, "Some Factors Controlling the Food Supply in China," *China Medical Journal* 25 (1921): 1–7.
22. Hartley Embrey and Tsou Ch'ing Wang, "Analysis of Some Chinese Foods," *China Medical Journal* 35 (1921): 247–57.
23. W. H. Adolph and P. C. Kiang, "The Nutritive Value of Soy Bean Products," *China Medical Journal* 34 (1920): 268–75; William H. Adolph, "Diet Studies in Shantung," *China Medical Journal* 37 (1923): 1013–19.
24. Thus the journal regularly reprints summaries of Western medical essays such as one taken from the *Berliner Klinische Wochenschrift* of March, 1914 advocating "cream and bed rest." *China Medical Journal* 29 (1915): 419–20.
25. Jean I. Dow, "Maternity Famine Relief," *China Medical Journal* 36 (1922): 59–67.
26. Letter to the editor by Sargent, "The Trade in Chinese Children," *China Medical Journal* 34 (1920): 695.
27. Thus in an editorial "Relation of Oriental Diet to Disease," *China Medical Journal* 38 (1924): 834–36 the concern is about diseases ranging from appendicitis to gall stones to cancer.
28. J.-P. Beaude, "OBESITE," in J.-P. Beaude, ed., *Dictionnaire de médecine usuelle à l'usage des gens du monde* (Paris : Didier, 1849), 2: 529–30.
29. Rousselot de Surgy, *Mélanges intéressans et curieux* (Paris : Lacombe, 1766), 4: 190.
30. Frederic W. Farrar, "Aptitudes of Races," *Transactions of the Ethnological Society of London*, 1867, 5: 115–26, here 124.
31. Arthur de Gobineau, *Essai sur l'inégalité des races humaines* (Paris: Librairie de Firmin Didot Frères, 1853), 1: 352.
32. Thomas King Chambers, "On The Pathology of Obesity," *Boston Medical and Surgical Journal* 43 (1851): 9–16.
33. J. Richardson Parke, *Human Sexuality: A Medico Literary Treatise* (Philadelphia: Spinoza Professional Publishing Company, 1912), 74.
34. Jefferys and Maxwell, *Diseases of China*, 320.
35. Thomas B. Futcher "Diabetes Mellitus And Ixsipidus," in William Osler, ed., *Modern Medicine: Its Theory And Practice* (Philadelphia and New York: Lea & Febiger, 1914). 1: 674–728, here 1: 674–5.
36. Osler, *Modern Medicine*, 751.
37. Quoted in Vivienne Lo and Penelope Barrett, "Cooking Up Fine Remedies: On the Culinary Aesthetic in a Sixteenth-century *Materia Medica*," *Medical History* 49 (2005): 395–422, here 417.
38. James L. Watson, *Food as Lens*, 208.
39. Wang Dungen "Reforming the Human Body" ("Renti Gailiang"), *Shenbao Ziyoutan* (29 August 1911: Tuesday), 3.

40. Mao Zedong, "A Study of Physical Education" (April, 1917), in *Mao's Road to Power: Revolutionary Writings 1912–1949*, ed., Stuart R. Schram, 5 vols. (Armonk, NY: M.E. Sharpe, 1992–1999), 1(1992): 113–127.
41. James L. Watson, *Food as Lens*, 208.
42. Shuhui and Weiseng, "On Obesity" ("Lun Feipang Zhi Bing"), *Funu Shibao [Women's Newspaper]* 10 (April, 1913), 26–28.
43. Wilhelm Ebstein, *Die Fettleibigkeit (Corpulenz) und ihre Behandlung nach physiologischen Grundstätzen*, 6th ed. (Wiesbaden: J. F. Bergmann, 1884), 10.
44. Dai Zuo, "Keep the Body Slim" ("Jianshou Ja"), *Jiatingzahi [Family Magazine]* 3 (1922), 1–4, here p. 1.
45. W. S. Hedley, *Therapeutic Electricity and Practical Muscle Testing* (Philadelphia: P. Blakiston's Son and Co., 1900), 209–10.
46. Zhou Zhenyu, "The Cause and Danger of Female Obesity," ("Funu Feipang De Yuanyin He Haichu"), *Xin Nuxing [The New Woman]* 1(1926), 42–45. Published in Shanghai, this journal had a reputation for its views on sexuality and health.
47. Anonymous, "What causes Obesity?" *Journal of the American Medical Association* (September 27, 1924): 1003.
48. Qi Hui, "Tragedy at the Dinner Table" ("Canzhuoshang De Beiju"), Liangyou 167 (June 1941), unpaged.
49. Sander L. Gilman, *Obesity: The Biography* (Oxford: Oxford University Press, 2010).
50. K. Day, M. Alfonzo, Y. Chen, Z. Guo, K. K. Lee, "Overweight, Obesity, and Inactivity and Urban Design in Rapidly Growing Chinese Cities. [Review]" *Health & Place* 21 (2013): 29–38
51. Y. Gao, S. Griffiths, E. Y. Y. Chan, "Community-based Interventions to Reduce Overweight and Obesity in China: A Systematic review of the Chinese and English Literature," *Journal of Public Health* (Oxford) 30 (2008): 436–448.
52. B.M. Popkin, "Will China's Nutrition Transition Overwhelm Its Health Care System and Slow Economic Growth?" *Health Affairs* 27 (4) (2008): 1064–1076.
53. Y.F. Wu, G.S. Ma, Y.H. Hu, Y.P. Li, X. Li, Z.H. Lui, C.M. Chen, L.Z. Kong, "The Current Prevalence of Body Overweight and Obesity in China: Data from The China National Nutrition and Health Survey," *Zhonghua Yu Fang Yi Xue Za* Zhi 39 (5) (2005): 319–320.
54. D. Qiu, X. Guo, J. Duan, L. Yang, N. Sakamoto, "Body mass index for Children aged 6–18 years in Beijing, China," *Annals of Human Biology*. 40 (2013): 301–8.
55. James A. Levine, "Obesity in China: Causes and Solutions," *Chinese Medical Journal* 121(2008): 1043–1050.
56. See Shannon Henson, "Obama's Launch Fight Against Childhood Obesity, Law360.com, February 9, 2010, http://www.law360.com/articles/148661/obamas-launch-fight-against-childhood-obesity (accessed November 19, 2013); Lynn Sweet, "Michelle Obama's remarks at 'Let's Move' launch. Prepared text," *Chicago Sun Times*, February 9, 2010, http://blogs.suntimes.com/sweet/2010/02/michelle_obamas_remarks_at_let.html (accessed November 12, 2013).
57. Brenda Major, Jeffrey Hunger, Debra Bunyan, Carol Miller, "The Ironic Effects of Weight Stigma," *Journal of Experimental Social Psychology* 51 (2014): 74–80, here 75.

Questions

Define "obesity."

What is a BMI?

How universal are the measurements of obesity?

What is an epidemic?

How is obesity understood in non-Western cultures?

Is obesity in China today different from obesity in the West?

What function does obesity have in the rethinking of what is modern in China as well as in the West?

Case Five

Seeing Pain

Problems: How do we know someone is in pain? Our bodies constantly express meaning. Our faces reflect those meanings. Are these meanings preprogrammed in our body and psyche, or do we project our reading of the interior life of other people on to their bodies? Pain tests the limits of these questions: Is pain literally written on their faces because of what we are experiencing, or is that experience and our understanding and expression of it determined by many other factors?

What Is Seeing in Medicine?

There is a sense within the health sciences that representations in medicine have to be mimetic to work. Representing the world—for instance, through the production of an X-ray of a human body—is a function of training to see accurately rather than an artifact of perception. When you look at an X-ray, the X-ray represents a real body, and the meaning of that image is fixed no matter who looks at the X-ray. It is clear that actual practice in medicine seems to undermine these claims that mimesis is a necessary aspect of the practice of medicine. Medical students are taught interpretation, and there is a constant, ongoing correction of the reading attached to images such as X-rays both in the moment and over time. The study of representations of the body is part of a debate about the possibility of "seeing the body" in an unmediated manner in medicine and in the humanities. Today's new functionalism in science seems to have moved toward stressing the "real" aspects of representing the body, in ways that are questioned by the very premises of theories of representation in the humanities. Medical science has returned to viewing representations of the body—whether through brain images or otherwise—as objective, and the disciplines of, by turns, neuroscience, evolutionary biology, and psychology as the single, unambiguous pathway to reading these representations without much attention to who sees and what is claimed to be seen.

This tension between objective scientific reality and a mediated sense of reality has existed, at least in Western thought, from the ancient world. Michel Foucault, in *The Order of Things* (1966), argues that the classical world saw representation as tied to experience and that only in modernity (which for him begins in the seventeenth century) was there the growing assumption that representations follow in complex ways their own rules and may or may not have any relationship to the experienced world.[1] Foucault also recognized that these rules that define the episteme change over time and from system to system of representation. David Morris argues, following Foucault, that by the eighteenth century, the interiority of pain was a "new way of seeing and of speaking" about pain.[2] Yet the belief was one that was understood as coming from an empirical point of view. There was a way of understanding the interior process of the body in an objective manner, though the clinical gaze.[3]

Certainly the problem of "seeing the body" is one that haunts medicine beginning with the Greeks. Greek medicine looks at the body, correlates the signs and symptoms found there and their expression with pathologies within the body. The physician Hippocrates (or at least the Hippocratic corpus) states that physicians must ask the patient about their status as well as observe the patient's body. What is learned is the basis for all diagnosis:

> When you examine the patient, inquire into all particulars; first how the head is . . . then examine if the hypochondrium and sides be free of pain, for . . . If there be pain in the side, and along with the pain either cough, tormina or bellyache, the bowels should be opened with clysters. . . . The physician should ascertain whether the patient be apt to faint when he is raised up, and whether his breathing is free; and examine the discharges from the bowels. . . . Attention should also be paid to the hands . . . and observe the nostrils . . . if the tongue be rough, and if there be swoonings, it is likely to be a remission of fever.[4]

There is no question that observing, including observing the fleeting physiognomy of illness, is the core of differential diagnosis in Greek (and later Roman) medicine. And so it should be, says modern medicine. We believe that we know intuitively what a healthy expression is and thus are attuned to the face of illness. Such awareness captures a wide range of expressions of illness and their manifestations. The one I wish to focus on in this chapter is that human experience of illness evoked by Hippocrates, the experience of pain. Pain features prominently in historical accounts of the visible and felt experience of illness and in recent debates about the representation of the body. Therefore, pain provides an excellent case study for exploring the historical and cultural meaning-making practices that construct healthy, ill, or "pained" bodies over time.

Can You See Pain? NO

One of the most remarkable factors in any medical discussion of pain, at least from the Enlightenment to the present, is the contradictory assumption of its immeasurability coupled with the claim of its innate visibility.[5] There is the view that scales of pain are by definition subjective, even within self-reporting pain scales (examples include the Numerical Rating Scale [NRS-11, NRS-101]; Visual Analog Scale; and Brief Pain Inventory, among others) that are now used to measure pain. Doctors have grappled with the inherently subjective nature of pain over the past half-century, as in this editorial from *The Lancet* in 1940:

> When the little girl said tearfully to her sister, "My toothache is worse than your toothache" she put her finger on the crux of the matter; for who shall say her nay? Pain is one of the phenomena that defy measurement, so many are the variables. Some will maintain that there is a wealth of diagnostic information contained in terms commonly applied to pain: gnawing, aching, pricking, stabbing, boring, tingling, cutting, shooting, starting, cramping, agonising, oppressive, bearing down, and many others; and the practitioner may never get the help from his scientific colleagues which will enable him to be more precise.[6]

But the subjectivity of pain is even more recently described as an artifact, not only of the patient's comprehension of pain, but equally a reflex of those attempting to measure pain through whatever scale is applied: "How a physician thinks about pain affects the way in which he or she assesses a patient who presents with pain."[7] Not only is the patient's account of their pain subjective, but so is the reception of their account by the physician. It is evident that character plays a major role in reporting pain. People are, following Riding and Cheema's dichotomy of "cognitive styles," either "levelers" or "sharpeners."[8] Some understate for personal, cultural, or perhaps even physiological reasons the intensity of their pain; others exaggerate it ("This is the *worst* pain I've ever had!"). In addition the context of the questioner/examiner always plays a major role in self-reporting of cognitive style.[9] But few self-reporting scales build this complexity into its evaluation.

Such descriptive representation of pain is not truly measurable even as medical science begins to attempt to measure pain because:

> Progress in measurement has been slow because pain is a complex perceptual experience that can be quantified only indirectly. Since pain has been operationalized in different ways in animal, human laboratory and clinical arenas of investigation the integration of knowledge across studies has been limited. The last decade has witnessed considerable innovation in pain measurement. . . .[10]

The notion that pain has objective, visual clues in other higher mammals[11] has been dismissed by researchers who find the human/animal analogy of visibility faulty:

> [Yet] many of the reflexes measured in animals are not found in man and this makes it difficult to draw strong, clinically relevant conclusions from experimental observations. The jaw opening reflex observed when dogs or cats are subjected to dental stimulation is not seen in the human although an inhibition of jaw closing muscles occurs. No human analogy to the tail flick response can be found, and human withdrawal latency when a hand is placed on a heated plate is vastly different from that of animals. Few investigators would agree with Vyklicky that the rodent writhing response captures the essence of the human experience of visceral pain.[12]

Animal models are different from human experiences, it is argued, but as is often the case humans project their own subjective experiences of pain into specific animal responses and see analogies between animals who appear to be in pain and their own expression of pain. (Perhaps, one can add here, that given our understanding of "pain," human beings can experience pain in ways that other mammals cannot in that not all physical pain may have a physical cause—but more about that later.)

If human beings find it difficult if not impossible to judge pain, then perhaps the problem is one of the limits of human apperception. In 2104 researchers at San Diego, Toronto, and Buffalo claimed that computers trained in facial recognition had a much better rate of differentiating between simulated expressions of pain and the real thing. Plunging their subject's arm in ice water, they measured the computer evaluation of these expressions against "deceptive facial signals" of the same subjects who had dipped their arms in warm water. Human evaluators could judge correctly whether the water was warm or cold only 55 percent of the time, while computers with self-correcting facial recognition software got it right 85 percent of the time.[13] Does this mean that there is an innate pain response from the subcortical region of the brain, only poorly mimicked by the cortical motor system that controls voluntary expression? Or does it mean that the computer over time learns to recognize the complexity of expression rather than its mere mimicry, a complexity that could have a wide range of meanings. Here "pain" is the label for a part of that complex of facial muscular expression that is possible in response to stimulus. In different cultures could the computer just as quickly learn to recognize different patterns of expressions of real rather than feigned pain? Is pain visible to computers in a way that it is not to human beings since people, even trained observers, are relatively poor judges of the nuances of expression?

Can You See Pain? YES

There are those, however, who claim quite the opposite: that there is a scientific, universal objective expression of pain that can provide access to its quantification in all human beings but even more so in the new claims about judging children's pain. The attempt to quantify pain understood in this manner is reflected in the design and use of subjective Observer Rated Pain Scales such as: FACES Pain Scale – Revised; CRIES Pain Scale for neonatal health care; Coloured Analogue Scale, FLACC Scale. These scientists agree with those who see any sort of self-measurement as difficult, flawed, or impossible, as those in pain cannot adequately describe their own experiences:

> People in pain convey their distress to others through a remarkably rich variety of expressive actions. These may include verbal report, paralinguistic vocalizations, withdrawal reflexes, palliative behavior, and changes in facial expression. Most systematic descriptions of pain, whether observed in the clinic or in the natural environment, have been devoted to verbal report. Self-report has numerous advantages for pain assessment, including methodological simplicity, apparent direct access to qualities of subjective experience, and evidence of empirical validity, because self-report commonly varies with tissue pathology and is responsive to healing. On the other hand, self-report indexes of pain may often be inadequate. The impact of situational and contextual variables raises doubts concerning the validity of self-report as a direct index of experience. Self-report is subject to voluntary control and hence to faking. In addition, children and many adults do not have the verbal skills needed to convey their distress effectively. Nonverbal expression provides an alternative source of pain information that would be expected to supplement and complement self-report measures for a variety of reasons. There is evidence that the impact of pain displays on others may be mediated by qualities of nonverbal expression.[14]

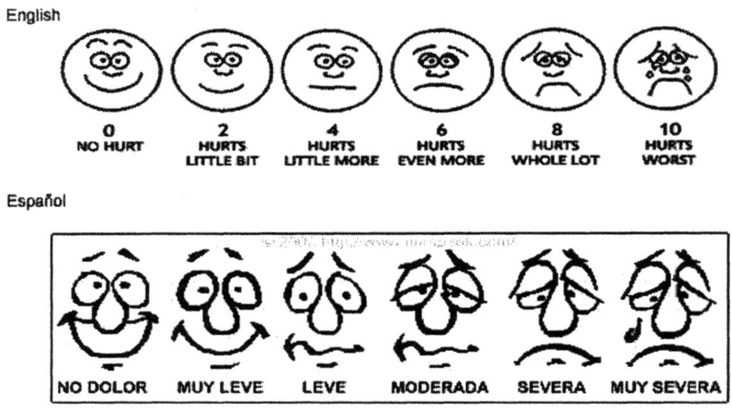

Figure 5.1. The Wong-Baker pain scale for adults and children three and up, in English and Spanish (private collection).

Only the scientist can claim any type of objective assessment of the patient's pain, and that assessment may be used to correct or negate any subjective statements about pain coming from a patient. Patients misconstrue; observers never do.

At the same time with the work of the psychologist Paul Ekman and his collaborators in the 1970s (and their Facial Expression; Awareness; Compassion; Emotions or F.A.C.E.S. project) the idea that the emotions can be seen and catalogued by trained observers through a catalogue of their visual expressions became a commonplace. Ekman's initial core emotions were Anger, Disgust, Fear, Happiness, Sadness, and Surprise; this list was substantially augmented later.[15] Pain, too, is to be seen and therefore measured, even if pain is not one of Ekman's primary states of emotion:

> Is there a consistent set of changes that occur in facial expression when pain occurs, regardless of the nature of the pain involved? . . . [is it] possible to discriminate spontaneous from deliberate pain expressions on the basis of facial action? . . . Whether the topography of facial behavior changes when people try to suppress or exaggerate the expression of pain. . . . When pain is expressed some four facial actions are likely to occur. The various analyses reported in the study support the assertion that the actions are cohesive, related to pain experience, and may properly be described as a "pain expression." . . . There maybe a universal expression of pain.[16]

The "face of pain" seems to be an objective reality whatever the motivation of the sufferer and, perhaps, whatever their cultural location.

Specific actions of the muscles of the face occur with pain, and these are observable, recordable, analyzable, and irrefutable.

Ekman's work was reinforced, if not based on, the claims of the American psychologist Silvan S. Tomkins, who argued that each emotion was physiologically different from all others and had universal, identifiable facial expressions. For Tomkins our responses to emotions were automatically triggered on the subcortical level.[17] These expressions were independent of any human thought or cultural intention. Tomkins's work began the modern study of facial expression and "provided the list of so-called basic emotions that, with minor modifications, stands today."[18] He also underpinned his claims with specific experimental evidence that emotions could be absolutely read from facial expression. As Ekman wrote, "Tomkins ... provided a theoretical rationale for studying the face as a means of learning about personality and emotion. He also showed that observers could obtain a very high agreement in judging emotion if the facial expressions were carefully selected to show what he believes are the innate facial affects."[19] This leads Ekman to the claim that such recognition is preprogrammed in each of us and not learned.

Underlying such claims are the findings of linguistics that other semantic fields in addition to articulated speech are part of the totality of communication. Gesture and expression (facial as well as bodily) are an intrinsic part of communication. Both are seen as hardwired in the development of the brain as part of a physiology of expression. In the case of pain, the body speaks more honestly than does the patient, as its communication is understood as unmediated and unmistakable (at least to the trained observer):

> The facial expression of pain has recently attracted considerable interest in experimental and clinical research based on an increasing awareness that it supports the communication of pain as a second signal system besides the verbal one. In line with this, facial activity provides the possibility to develop pain assessment tools in individuals with limited abilities to communicate pain verbally (e.g. newborns, individuals with pronounced cognitive impairments and dementia). An early and very important observation as regards facial responses associated with pain, was that there is a subset of key facial muscle movements that are displayed consistently across different pain modalities. This subset of pain-relevant facial responses includes brow lowering, orbit tightening, levator contraction and eye closure. Although there is convergent evidence that these facial responses constitute the core of the "pain face," there are also other

> facial muscle movements that have frequently been observed in the context of pain.[20]

The "pain face" can be read, can be the basis for evaluation, and can provide the sort of instrument for representing the body that self-reporting can never be. Indeed, the lines between self-assessment and seeing are often blurred, as can be seen in The Wong Baker Faces Pain Scale, developed by the pediatric nurses Donna Wong and Connie M. Baker in 1981. The scale uses the Ekman F.A.C.E.S scale for self-assessment, and we can assume that the patient is not staring at a mirror but rather reporting the way they imagine their pain to look.

Empathy

The dichotomy between immeasurability and perception is not only a feature of the medical literature. The question of immediate response to pain as a philosophical problem of empathy (what Ekman and the Dalai Lama call "compassion") demands the unmediated "seeing" of a subjective category.[21] Even Elaine Scarry, whose seminal book, *The Body in Pain*, first raised the question of pain as a social phenomenon for the humanist, seems to see pain's perception as unmediated:

> If one imagines one human being seeing another human being in pain, one human being perceiving in another discomfort and in the same moment wishing the other to be relieved of the discomfort, something in that faction of a second is occurring inside the first person's brain involving the complex action of many neurons that is, importantly, not just a perception of actuality (the second person's pain) but an alteration of actuality (for embedded in the perception is the sorrow that it is so, the wish that it were otherwise).[22]

Pain can, indeed, must be seen for us to be empathic to those who are in "discomfort."

Those who argue against such reductionism of the act of seeing (even with its concomitant empathy) call for our awareness that seeing is always a form of cultural mediation, with so-called display rules developed within any given culture. Psychologists such as Alan J. Fridlund and James A. Russell see an absolute link between pure experience of emotions and its physiological expression as unsupportable.[23] They argue, against the theories put forth by Ekman et al., that cultural rules govern how emotions are expressed, but there is no question that they are expressed and that they are always expressed. Thus Russell notes in

1994 that pain is *not* one of the "basic" emotions to which the observers of emotion, such as Ekman, have reduced facial expression:

> Facial movements include not just the 7 ± 2 "facial expressions of emotion," but laughs, pouts, yawns, winces, grimaces, and all manner of actions difficult to describe. In our culture, people use facial cues to infer sleepiness, relaxation, puzzlement, confusion, pain, boredom, interest, attention, and other states besides seven "basic" emotions. An understanding of facial expressions would be helped by integrating studies over the full range of facial movements and inferences from them. . . . Rather than ask whether a given culture agrees with one preformulated hypothesis, we might more usefully ask how members of that culture conceptualize emotions and facial behavior. There may be no short cut to obtaining the needed information. Although the task is great, what we know about the peoples of different cultures suggests that carrying it out will be fascinating.[24]

But "seen" pain must be uniform across cultures since the "black box" of the expression of emotions is hardwired, even if their specific expressions may not be.

The nuances of representing the body are determined in this view by culture, but the body will express a range of emotions even if their expression differs from culture to culture and time to time. This is an evolutionary fact: only the expression and perception of states such as pain (and its construction from other forms of emotional expression) are culturally determined. This view underpins the work on the so-called "praecox feeling" first undertaken by the Dutch phenomenological psychiatrist Henricus Cornelius Rümke in the 1940s.[25] Experienced mental health professionals who work with the mentally ill come to be able to "intuitively" distinguish them from healthy people, or so it has been claimed. In doing so they lose any sense of "empathy" with the patient. What is actually "seen" are the subtle shifts in nonverbal communication that occur in certain manifestations of the schizophrenias. Specifically, physicians learn that empathic identification with such patients does not elicit any appropriate affective response. After having seen enough patients, one becomes subconsciously attuned to this expression. Neither the expression of the illness nor its perception is in any way hardwired. It is a purely learned awareness, and it may even be a learned awareness not of a specific pathological presentation of schizophrenia but of the cultural patterns by which those suffering from mental illness can express their symptoms.[26]

Now, both the schools of Ekman and Russell are biologically grounded. Pain and its expression are reflections of the workings of a black box of emotions. The former assumes that the categories of expression are fixed and are mimetic of an underlying scale of emotions; the latter sees these fixed forms as culturally selected. The scale of the expression of pain in the former is fixed because of the relationship between emotion and expression; in the latter, the scale is fixed because a given culture has selected from among the widest potential means of expression and underlying emotions those that articulate pain best. The true alternative to both would be that we are born with facial muscles, that these muscles develop over time as we learn the scale of emotions in our world. A radical cultural theory of pain would see our adult projection of pain into the actions of the infant as a loop by which we train infants to express pain.

Can You See Pain in the Brain?

We might imagine that the most recent advances in medical imaging would resolve this conundrum, but an fMRI today is no more a simple reflection of underlying realities than were X-rays a century ago. While there has been a great deal of work done on pain and its representation in images of the living brain, most of it has been aimed as researching the nature of brain responses to painful stimuli rather than developing a diagnostic tool for representing pain.[27] Recent studies have attempted to distinguish the psychological impact of expectation of pain—how individuals react to the belief that they will feel pain in the future—on its mental representation and studies of brain scans now evoke the "biopsychosocial" nature of pain.[28] The problem even with such sophisticated studies that take the totality of experience under consideration is that they assume a more or less uniform representation of complex mental states in fMRIs. Thus one recent study makes an attempt to tease out differences in pain sensitivity based on self-reporting. The researchers sought objective criteria (as does the Wong Baker test) to measure the accuracy of such self-reporting. They claim that there are objective correlatives between the image of complex brain activation and the self-reporting of levels of pain and that this correlation could be used to determine levels of medical intervention. They register differences in individual response to identical stimuli but postulate that these differences may well lie in earlier experience of pain, the emotional state of the subject as well as the expectations of pain.[29] Yet the idea that one can "see" the totality of such experiences relative one to the other seems illogical. If individuals have a wide range of experiences that shape their own sense of what is painful, and if these experiences are diverse and are located in complex ways in the brain, each scan must be unique and thus would tell us even less than asking "how much does it hurt?"

Even the question of empathy to pain has been explored using brain scans. This one recent study claims that when children see an image of a person in pain, the portions of their brain that would have registered that pain on an fMRI scan respond. When the children see a person intentionally hurt, portions of the brain associated with "moral reasoning" are also activated.[30] The idea that empathy means an affective identification with the experience of the pain of another based on one's own prior experience of pain demands some qualification. Do all individuals respond to all manifestations of pain in the same way? Certainly a "biopsychosocial" model would argue that they do not. At least one study thinks that one needs to already have had some type of empathic relationship with the person in pain.

> Our ability to have an experience of another's pain is characteristic of empathy. Using functional imaging, we assessed brain activity while volunteers experienced a painful stimulus and compared it to that elicited when they observed a signal indicating that their loved one—present in the same room—was receiving a similar pain stimulus.[31]

This claim evokes echoes of the infamous (and now oft rebutted) Stanley Milgram experiment in which pain was inflicted on a third person while the "scientist" observed and ordered increasingly painful shocks. Here anonymity is replaced by emotional connection. Do we always respond as the researchers here indicted, and what is the nature of the brain coordinates for "moral reasoning"? Indeed, can we even through brain scans distinguish empathetic pain from the pain of a "broken heart"? At least one brain neuroimaging study claims to show that that the brain areas that are activated during the distress caused by social exclusion are also those activated during physical pain.[32]

All of these studies and a much wider range of brain scans representing "pain" in all of its multitudinous firms fall into the pattern of errors that earlier theories of pain entailed. They elide our Western, popular understanding of "pain" and "empathy." They do not attempt to ask how much of the very experience of "seeing" pain is formed by the cultures of pain in which each of us as individuals mature and which seem to each of us "natural." That such patterns would be found in the pain is obvious, as it is the brain that catalogues and records, for better or ill, such experiences. But as Eric Racine, Ofek Bar-Ilan, and Judy Illes noted in a major study of the popular reception of such studies, brain imaging experiments "can make a phenomenon uncritically real, objective or effective in the eyes of the public."[33] They described this phenomenon as "neuro-realism":

> Many occurrences of neuro-realism deal with the effectiveness of health-related procedures such as acupuncture. For example, "Patients have long reported that acupuncture helps relieve their pain, but scientists don't know why. Could it be an illusion? Now brain imaging technology has indicated that the perception of pain relief is accurate." Another headline: "A relatively new form of brain imaging provides visual proof that acupuncture alleviates pain."[34]

The underlying claim is that "the brain can't lie: brain scans reveal how you think and feel and even how you might behave.'"[35] Often such neuro-realism haunts the very science that is received by the public. This form of fantasy is the basis for much of the biological approaches to seeing pain. While it may be believed that brain imaging provides visual proof that certain interventions ameliorate pain, the simple reality is that only the subject can state whether pain has been relieved or not. And self-reporting is the slave to the context in all of its complexity in which the report is made and in which the individual experiences pain. All of the images of relief are useless unless the individual feels relief. And relief may have to do with experience of pain and its relief (as in a placebo) than in any mimetic representation of pain in the brain.

Thus we are struck by a conundrum: the more subjective pain is from the standpoint of the sufferer, the more objective it is from the standpoint of the observer, unless of course the observer too is subjective. "Seeing is believing" unless we don't believe in seeing. Or at least believe that seeing is unmediated.

A History of Seeing Pain

This problem is, not surprisingly, not a new one. Scientists in the Enlightenment came to doubt the efficacy of unmediated seeing in diagnosis.[36] How much of what we see is an artifact of who were are? This question is asked in detail by the American physician Benjamin Rush (1746–1813) in the eighteenth century:

> Physicians by reviewing the history of complaints from their patients will often have them exaggerated but by frequent visits you cannot

> be deceived. . . . Endeavor to get the history of the disease from the patient himself and do not interrupt him till he has finished as he will always give the best symptoms tho' he may give the worst causes. Begin to interrogate your patient. By how long he has been sick? When attacked and in what manner? What are the probable causes, former habits and dress; likewise the diet, etc., for a week before especially in acute diseases. . . . In chronic diseases enquire their complaints far back and the habits of life. . . . Pay attention to the phraseology of your patients, for the same ideas are frequently conveyed in different words. A pain in the precordia is called by an Englishman a pain in his stomach, by a Scotchman in his breasts, an Irishman in his heart and by a Southern man mighty poorly. Enquire of your patients the diseases of their ancestors, the age to which they lived and the remedies which relieved them. It is of consequence because there is a hereditary idiosyncrasies in some families. Patients often conceal the cause of their disease—therefore interrogate them particularly when you suspect intemperance as the cause of disease.[37]

Pain is for Rush the exemplary case of patient misunderstanding; only the physician trained in taking a history can comprehend it. The patient's language is insufficient or perhaps too local to communicate his/her experience. Culture articulates pain; one trained in observing the variations in its expression can interpret it.

It was the Scottish physician and anatomist Charles Bell (1774–1842) who put forth perhaps the clearest claim to representing bodily pain in his *Essays on The Anatomy of Expression in Painting* (1806), later republished as *Essays on The Anatomy and Philosophy of Expression* in 1824. Bell claimed that the very structure of the musculature of the face was solely present in order for man to expression emotions. Aimed at art students the task of his study was to provide them with the visual vocabulary of human expression generated by those muscles, including that of pain:

> In bodily pain the jaws are fixed and the teeth grind; the lips are drawn laterally, so as to expose the teeth and gums; the nostrils are distended to the utmost, and at the same time drawn up; the eyes are largely uncovered, and the eyebrows elevated; the face is turgid with blood, and the veins of the forehead and temples distended, the breath being suspended, and the descent of the blood from the head impeded. Much of the expression results from the strong action of the muscles closing the jaws, and the strong action and consequent stringiness of the cutaneous muscles of the neck R, plate II, which at the same time draws down the corner of the mouth.[38]

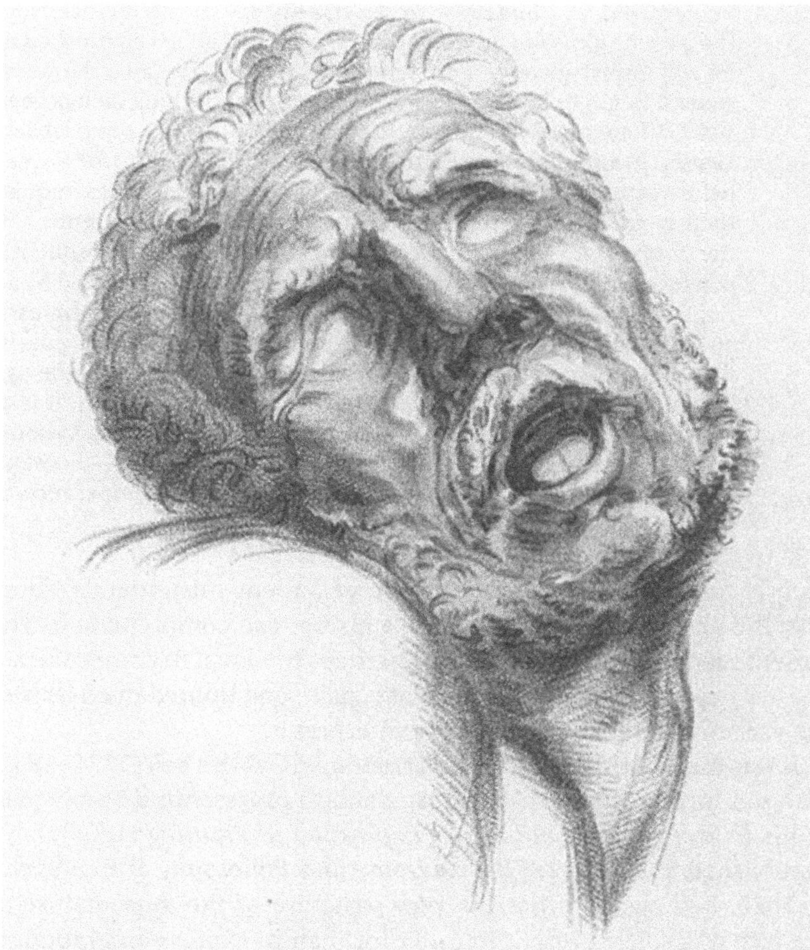

Figure 5.2. "Pain" from Charles Bell, *The Anatomy and Philosophy of Expression as Connected with the Fine Arts.* Third edition. (London: J. Murray, 1844).

Bell's claim is that such expression is both universal and mechanical. But Bell, prefiguring Scarry's understanding of empathy, also speaks of the internal state of the psyche that is readable through the transparency of the "face of pain." It is a readability that cannot be obfuscated or denied:

> In pain, the body is exerted to violent tension, and all the emotions and passions which are allied to pain, or have their origin and foundation in painful sensations, have distinctly this character in common, that there is tension, or a start into exertion, or tremor, the effect of universal and great excitement. It must at the same time be recollected, that all the passions of this class, some more immediately,

> others more indirectly, produce in the second stage a loss of tone, exhaustion, and debility, from over exertion. . . . Pain first rouses the faculties both of the body and of the mind, and from a dormant state gives us consciousness and real existence. It is bestowed upon us as a perpetual guard, forcing us to watch continually for the safety of the body and the preservation of life. From the expression of pain as a centre we may trace the indications of many of the mixed passions.[39]

Pain is both a safety mechanism to protect the body from damage, and its expression allows others to see our pain.

Bell's work is evoked by the most important scientist to deal with the visibility of pain. Charles Darwin (1809–1882), whose *The Expression of the Emotions in Man and Animals*, published in 1872, saw expression and its recognition as a means of the survival of the fittest. Darwin is seen by many contemporary scholars of emotions, such as Ekman, as their major precursor.[40] Darwin assumes animal analogies as evidence to prove the evolutionary origin of expressions, such as those of pain, counter too much of the contemporary work on expression discussed above. Darwin also refers back to Bell for his argument about seeing pain and continues Bell's argument in the 1870s.

> . . . the long-continued habit of attempting by struggling to escape from the cause of suffering—and the consciousness that voluntary muscular exertion relieves pain, have all probably concurred in giving a tendency to the most violent, almost convulsive, movements under extreme suffering; and such movements, including those of the vocal organs, are universally recognised as highly expressive of this condition.[41]

But like our contemporary "seers of pain" Darwin too relies on the response of the observer to document Bell's accuracy rather than simply relying on the scientist's observation:

> Sir C. Bell remarks that "horror is full of energy;" the body is in the utmost tension, not unnerved by "fear." It is, therefore, probable that horror would generally be accompanied by the strong contraction of the brows; but as fear is one of the elements, the eyes and mouth would be opened, and the eyebrows would be raised, as far as the antagonistic action of the corrugators permitted this movement. Duchenne has given a photograph of the same old man as before, with his eyes somewhat staring, the eyebrows partially raised, and at the same time strongly contracted, the mouth opened, and the platysma in action, all effected by the means of galvanism. He considers that the expression thus produced shows extreme terror with horrible

> pain or torture. A tortured man, as long as his sufferings allowed him to feel any dread for the future, would probably exhibit horror in an extreme degree. I have shown the original of this photograph to twenty-three persons of both sexes and various ages; and thirteen immediately answered horror, great pain, torture, or agony; three answered extreme fright; so that sixteen answered nearly in accordance with Duchenne's belief.[42]

Darwin draws on Bell's theory but on the photographs of Guillaume-Benjamin-Amand Duchenne (known as de Boulogne) (1806–1875) as Bell's romantic engravings were clearly "art," while Duchenne's photographs gave Darwin (he believed) an unmediated representation of pain.[43] As is clear today, Duchenne's photographs, posed by well-known actors of the day, reflected less a true expression of pain but rather the musculature needed to create the impression of pain for the theatrical audience.[44] Darwin's idea of pain as readable in the human physiognomy is dependent on the consensus of observer and patient as to how pain is to be legibly expressed. Further, Darwin draws what is expressed into question. Bell believes individuals have to experience "real" (i.e., physical) pain to have the face of pain; for Darwin it is the expression of the musculature in pain—mirroring that in other animals—that shows the continuity of pain expression across species. Darwin understands, following Duchenne, that one does not have to experience pain to express it.

Darwin acknowledges that the *belief* that one is in physical pain is equivalent to being in pain. He approached James Crichton Browne, director of the West Riding Asylum and a passionate photographer, for images of the mentally ill.[45] In turn in 1869, Charles Darwin sent him a copy of Duchenne's studies of the electrical stimulation of the facial nerves. Darwin incorporated Crichton Browne's photographs of the mentally ill into his study:

> . . . I begged for information from Dr. Crichton Browne with respect to the insane. He states in answer that he has repeatedly seen their hair erected under the influence of sudden and extreme terror. For instance, it is occasionally necessary to inject morphia under the skin of an insane woman, who dreads the operation extremely, though it causes very little pain; for she believes that poison is being introduced into her system, and that her bones will be softened, and her flesh turned into dust. She becomes deadly pale; her limbs are stiffened by a sort of tetanic spasm, and her hair is partially erected on the front of the head.[46]

Unlike in Bell's study, the very connection between the observable external state of the body and the internal source of that state is drawn into question. Pain may be imagined and be expressed as accurately as if it were "actually" experienced.

An Alternative View

It would seem that the question of an unmediated representation of pain, if one reads Paul Ekman, is uncontested after Darwin, yet it is in the work of Sigmund Freud (1856–1939) that Darwin's idea of pain as physical and psychic is confronted in the early 1890s. His teacher, Theodor Meynert, had made reference in his textbook of 1884 to Darwin's theory of expression as the "through such movements as are involved in expression we obtain a clue to the inner life of others."[47] Freud, who remained a classic Darwinian his entire creative life, is thus early trained to "see" those afflicted with pain. When he goes to Paris in 1885 to study with the neurologist Jean-Martin Charcot, he is confronted with a scientist who relies on the photograph to document states of psychic (rather than physical) pain and has his view that "seeing is believing" reified.[48] In an essay in 1890 entitled "Psychical (or Mental) Treatment" he writes in a pure Darwinian way that:

> The commonest, everyday example of the mind's action on the body, and one that is to be observed in everyone, is offered by what is known as the "expression of the emotions." A man's states of mind are manifested, almost without exception, in the tensions and relaxations of his facial muscles, in the adaptations of his eyes, in the amount of blood in the vessels of his skin, in the modifications in his vocal apparatus and in the movements of his limbs and in particular of his hands. These concomitant physical changes are for the most part of no advantage to the person concerned; on the contrary, they often stand in his way if he wishes to conceal his mental processes from other people. But they serve these other people as trustworthy indications from which his mental processes can be inferred and in which more confidence can be placed than in any simultaneous verbal expressions that may be made deliberately.[49]

At the same time Freud was obsessed with the phenomenon of physical pain and its amelioration, experimenting with cocaine as a local anesthetic in the early 1880s.

But it was only after he returned to Vienna from Paris in the mid-1880s that he became fascinated by Darwin's claim that one can have physical pain brought about by a psychological cause as there may be "a 'symbolic' relation between the precipitating cause and the pathological phenomenon—a relation such as healthy people form in dreams. For instance, a neuralgia may follow upon mental pain or vomiting upon a feeling of moral disgust."[50] Not a lesion in the nervous system, which could not be seen by contemporary means of visualization, as Charcot claimed, but underlying psychic causes could also cause physical pain. And here we can return to the question asked earlier: what happens when not all physical pain has a physical cause? Conversion disorders translate psychic symptoms into physical ones, including pain. But, as Freud comes to understand that such physical pain as caused by psychic mechanisms such as repression is rarely linked to a specific form of remembering as representation. It is not simply the direct translation of one (the cause) into the other (the symptom), and thus such pain is quite different from the idea of the symptom as developed in the *Studies on Hysteria* (1895) (where the anxiety surrounding seeing a dog drinking from a glass becomes expressed by a patient as the inability to swallow). Physical pain becomes for Freud a clinical "compass" to understand more complex psychic mechanisms.

While Freud is anxious at the time that focusing on the psychological function of pain may cause him to overlook some physical cause, as he recounts in his "Dream of Irma's Injection" in the *Interpretation of Dreams.*[51] Yet he applies Darwin to his cases of hysteria as in the case of "Emmy von N":

> Some of the striking motor phenomena exhibited by Frau von N. were simply an expression of the emotions and could easily be recognized in that light. Thus, the way in which she stretched her hands in front of her with her fingers spread out and crooked expressed horror, and similarly her facial play. This, of course, was a more lively and uninhibited way of expressing her emotions than was usual with women of her education and race. Indeed, she herself was restrained, almost stiff in her expressive movements when she was not in a hysterical state. Others of her motor symptoms were, according to herself, directly related to her pains. She played restlessly with her fingers (1888) or rubbed her hands against one another (1889) so as to prevent herself from screaming. This reason reminds one forcibly of one of the principles laid down by Darwin to explain the expression of the emotions—the principle of the overflow of excitation, which accounts, for instance, for dogs wagging their tails.[52]

By this point Freud had broken with Charcot's understanding of representation, dismissing him in 1893 as "not unduly reflective, not a thinker: he had the nature of an artist—he was, as he himself said, a 'visuel', a man who sees. Here is what he himself told us about his method of working. He used to look again and again at the things he did not understand, to deepen his impression of them day by day, till suddenly an understanding of them dawned on him."[53] But, of course, this was a false "seeing," and Freud replaces seeing in his mode of representation (and therapy) with listening. Yet it is also the case that his idea of representing psychic pain is one still very much in the Darwinian mode, with an added understanding of the deformation of symptoms in their very expression:

> What could be more probable than that the figure of speech "swallowing something", which we use in talking of an insult to which no rejoinder has been made, did in fact originate from the innervatory sensations which arise in the pharynx when we refrain from speaking and prevent ourselves from reacting to the insult? All these sensations and innervations belong to the field of "the expression of the emotions", which, as Darwin has taught us, consists of actions which originally had a meaning and served a purpose. These may now for the most part have become so much weakened that the expression of them in words seems to us only to be a figurative picture of them, whereas in all probability the description was once meant literally; and hysteria is right in restoring the original meaning of the words in depicting its unusually strong innervations.[54]

Freud is able to depart from a strict reading of the Darwin's model to understand that the representation of pain may well be tangentially to a "real experience," which is, of course, Darwin's own view on his analysis of mental illness and pain.

While Freud initially believes that listening is a means of representation that is objective, he eventually becomes aware of counter-transference that the therapist too is subjective in listening in the analytic situation. As he writes in 1928 to Sándor Ferenczi concerning the question of counter-transference:

> All those who have no tact will see in this a justification of arbitrariness, i.e., of the subjective factor, i.e., of the influence of one's own unrestrained complexes. What we undertake in reality is a weighing out, which remains mostly preconscious, of the various reactions that we expect from our interventions, in the process of which it is first and foremost a matter of the quantitative assessment of the dynamic factors in the situation. Rules for these measurements can naturally not be made; the analyst's experience and normality will have to be

> the decisive factors. But one should thus divest "tact" of its mystical character for beginners.[55]

To this we should certainly add the need to divest representations and their observation of all sort of their "mystical character." But also, following Freud, we should be very careful of "empathy" on the part of the observer, for empathy (that force that thinkers from Bell to Scarry associate with seeing pain) may well be a reflection, not of our comprehension of the Other, but of our own projection onto the Other. Seeing may be the creation of a false empathy of the Other's pain.

Seeing pain has a history. It also has a practice in the science of medicine, both ancient and modern. Medicine "sees" pain, or at least its representations. But how this act of seeing is understood is part of any epistemology of medicine. Pain becomes a vital site for the meanings attached to conflicting systems of representation. Karen Barad in her *Meeting the Universe Halfway* dismisses the "Cartesian distinction between objects and agencies of observation" to suggest that "measurement practices are an ineliminable part of the results obtained."[56] Pain measurement of all types demands an act (self-reporting or observation or both) that is part of the boundaries drawn, so that "method, measurement, description, interpretation, epistemology, and ontology are not separable considerations."[57] If measurement cannot be separated from what is being measured, Barad concludes that "measured properties refer to phenomena."[58] More specifically, she says:

> I argue that phenomena are not the mere result of laboratory exercises engineered by human subjects; rather, *phenomena are differential patterns of mattering* ("diffraction patterns") produced through complex agential intra-actions of multiple material discursive practice or apparatuses of bodily production, where *apparatuses are not mere observing instruments but boundary drawing practices—specific material (re)configurings of the world—which come to matter.*[59]

Pain is just such a "diffraction pattern" which is bounded as a representation by its very examination.

The debates about pain and its expression are ongoing. In the end, however, these debates are about the most efficient manner of representing the body. How one sees and understands the body is an artifact of the theories one has about the very nature of seeing. Dealing with categories such as pain illustrate that even what may seem obvious in representing the body demand complicated means of understanding the very nature of representation and its claims.

Notes

1. Michel Foucault, *The Order of Things: An Archaeology of the Human Sciences.* (New York: Vintage, 1994).
2. David B. Morris, *The Culture of Pain* (Berkeley: University of California Press, 1993).
3. Ibid., 226.
4. Roy Porter, *The Greatest Benefit to Mankind: A Medical History of Humanity* (London: HarperCollins, 1997), here 61.
5. On this topic, see Jan Frans van Dijkhuizen, *Pain and Compassion in Early Modern English Literature and Culture* (New York: D.S. Brewer, 2012); Ronald D. Mann, ed. *The History of the Management of Pain: From Early Principles to Present Practice* (Carnforth, UK: Parthenon Pub. Group, 1988); Martin S. A. Pernick, *Calculus of Suffering: Pain, Professionalism, and Anesthesia in Nineteenth-Century America* (New York: Columbia University Press, 1985); Roselyne Rey, *History of Pain,* trans. Louise Elliott Wallace and J. A. and S. W. Cadden (Paris: La Découverte, 1993); Melanie Thernstrom, *The Pain Chronicles: Cures, Myths, Mysteries, Prayers, Diaries, Brain Scans, Healing, and the Science Of Suffering* (New York: Farrar, Straus and Giroux, 2010).
6. Anonymous, "The Measurement of Pain," *The Lancet* 236, no. 6102 (1940): 167.
7. Dennis C. Turk and Akiko Okifuji. "Assessment of Patients' Reporting of Pain: An Integrated Perspective," *The Lancet* 353, no. 9166 (1999): 1784–88, here 1784.
8. Richard Riding and Indra Cheema. "Cognitive Styles—An Overview and Integration," *Educational Psychology* 11.3 (1991): 193–215.
9. Ibid., 202.
10. C. R. Chapman, et al., "Pain Measurement: an Overview," *Pain* 22 (1985): 1–31, here 2.
11. D. B. Morton and P. H. M. Griffiths. "Guidelines on the Recognition of Pain, Distress and Discomfort in Experimental Animals and An Hypothesis for Assessment," *The Veterinary Record* 116 (April 1985): 431–436.
12. Chapman, 2.
13. Marian Stewart Bartlett, Gwen C. Littlewort, Mark G. Frank and Kang Lee. "Automatic Decoding of Facial Movements Reveals Deceptive Pain Expressions," *Current Biology* 24 (7) (2014): 738–43.
14. Kenneth D. Craig and Christopher J. Patrick. "Facial Expression During Induced Pain," *Journal of Personality and Social Psychology* 48 (1985): 1080–1091, here 1080.
15. Paul Ekman and Wallace V. Friesen. "The Repertoire of Nonverbal Behavior: Categories, Origins, Usage, and Coding," *Semiotica*, 1 (1969): 49–98; Paul Ekman and Wallace V. Friesen "Constants across Cultures in the Face And Emotion," *Journal of Personality and Social Psychology* 17 (1971): 124–19.
16. Kenneth M. Prkachin, "Facial Expressions of Pain: A Comparison across Modalities," in Paul Ekman, Erika L. Rosenberg, eds., *What the Face Reveals: Basic and Applied Studies of Spontaneous Expression Using the Facial Action Coding System (FACS)* (New York: Oxford University Press, 2005), 181–97; afterword: 198–202, here 202.
17. Ruth Leys, "The Turn to Affect: A Critique," *Critical Inquiry* 37 (2011): 434–72; response in *Critical Inquiry* 38 (2012): 882–891.

18. Alan J. Fridlund, *Human Facial Expression: An Evolutionary View* (San Diego: Academic Press, 1994), here 198.
19. Paul Ekman, "The Argument and Evidence about Universals in Facial Expressions of Emotion," in *Handbook of Social Psychopathology: Emotion and Social Behavior*, ed. H. Wagner and A. Manstead (New York: Wiley, 1989), here 145.
20. Miriam Kunz, Kenneth Prkachin, and Stefan Lautenbacher. "The Smile of Pain," *Pain* 145 (2009): 273–275, here 273.
21. The Dalai Lama and Paul Ekman. *Emotional Awareness: Overcoming the Obstacles to Psychological Balance and Compassion* (New York: New York Times Books, 2008).
22. Elaine Scarry, *The Body In Pain: The Making and Unmaking of the World* (New York: Oxford University Press, 1985), here 289.
23. Fridlund, *Human Facial Expression.*
24. James A. Russell, "Is there Universal Recognition of Emotion from Facial Expression? A Review of the Cross-Cultural Studies," *Psychological Bulletin* 115 (1994): 102–141, here 141.
25. H. C. Rümke, "The Nuclear Symptom of Schizophrenia and the Praecox Feeling," trans. Jan Neeleman. *History of Psychiatry* 1 (1990): 331–41.
26. Sander L. Gilman, "Why is Schizophrenia 'Bizarre': An Historical Essay in the Vocabulary of Psychiatry," *Journal of the History of the Behavioral Sciences* 19 (1983): 127–135.
27. P. Schweinhardt and M. C. Bushnell, "Pain Imaging in Health and Disease—How Far Have We Come?" *Journal of Clinical Investigations* 120 (November 2010): 3788–3797.
28. J. Kong, et al., "Expectancy and Treatment Interactions: A Dissociation between Acupuncture Analgesia and Expectancy Evoked Placebo Analgesia," *NeuroImage* 45 (April 2009): 940–949.
29. Christopher J. Starr, Timothy T. Houle, and Robert C. Coghill, "Psychological and Sensory Predictors of Experimental Thermal Pain: A Multifactorial Model," *Journal of Pain* 11, no. 12 (2010): 1394–1402.
30. Jean Decety, Kalina Michalska, and Yuko Aktsuki, "Who Caused the Pain? An fMRI Investigation of Empathy and Intentionality in Children," *Neuropsychologia* 46 (2008): 2607–2614.
31. Tania Singer, et al., "Empathy for Pain Involves the Affective but not Sensory Components of Pain," *Science* (February 2004): 1157–1162, here 1157.
32. Naomi I. Eisenberger, Matthew D. Lieberman, and Kipling D. Williams, "Does Rejection Hurt? An fMRI Study of Social Exclusion," *Science* (October 2003): 290–292.
33. Eric Racine, Ofek Bar-Ilan, and Judy Illes, "Science and Society: fMRI in the Public Eye," *Nature Reviews Neuroscience* 6 (February 2005): 159–164, here 160.
34. Ibid.
35. Ibid.
36. See Simon Richter, *Laocoon's Body and the Aesthetics of Pain: Winckelmann, Lessing, Herder, Moritz, Goethe.* (Detroit: Wayne State University Press, 1992).
37. Porter, *Greatest Benefit*, 257.
38. Charles Bell. *Essays on The Anatomy and Philosophy of Expression* (London: John Murray, 1824), here 96.

39. Ibid.
40. Paul Ekman, ed. *Darwin and Facial Expression: A Century of Research in Review* (New York: Academic Press, 1973).
41. Charles Darwin, *The Expression of the Emotions in Man and Animals* (London: John Murray, 1872), here 73.
42. Ibid., 305.
43. G. -B. Duchenne de Boulogne, *The Mechanism of Human Facial Expression (Studies in Emotion and Social Interaction)*, trans. R. Andrew Cuthbertson (Cambridge: Cambridge University Press, 1990,) here 60.
44. Sander L. Gilman, *Seeing the Insane: A Cultural History of Psychiatric Illustration* (New York: Wiley Interscience, 1982), here 164.
45. Ibid., 179.
46. Darwin, *Emotions*, 295.
47. Lucille B. Ritvo, *Darwin's Influence on Freud: A Tale of Two Sciences* (Yale University Press, New Haven, 1990).
48. Andrew Hodgkiss, *From Lesion to Metaphor: Chronic Pain In British, French And German Medical Writings, 1800–1914* (Amsterdam: Rodopi, 2000), here 64.
49. Sigmund Freud, *Standard Edition of the Complete Psychological Works of Sigmund Freud*, ed. and trans. James Strachey, Anna Freud, Alix Strachey, and Alan Tyson. 24 vols. London: Hogarth, 1955–74, cited as SE, here VII, 285.
50. Freud/Breuer, SE, *Hysteria*, Vol. II, 1.
51. Freud, SE, Vol. IV, 106.
52. Freud, SE, Vol. II, 90.
53. Freud, SE, Vol. III, 10.
54. Freud, SE, Vol. II, 180.
55. Sigmund Freud and Sándor Ferenczi. *The Correspondence of Sigmund Freud and Sándor Ferenczi.* Vol. III, 1920–1933, ed. Ernst Falzeder, Eva Brabant, with Patrizia Giampieri-Deutsch, trans. Peter Hoffer (Cambridge, MA: Harvard University Press, 2000), here 333.
56. Karen Barad, *Meeting the Universe Halfway: Quantum Physics and the Entanglement of Matter and Meaning* (Durham: Duke UP, 2007), here 120–121.
57. Ibid., 121.
58. Ibid., 197.
59. Ibid., 140, emphasis in original.

Questions

What is pain?

Who defines pain?

Is pain in the body? Is it in the mind?

What is psychic pain?

What do brain scans measure?

How does Charles Darwin understand the function of representations (such as photographs) as evidence for his theory of pain?

What do photographs actually document as evidence in the medical humanities?

Can you imagine an illness separate from how it is understood in its cultural context?

Case Six

Madness as a Disability

Problems: How does society imagine mental illness? Does this shift radially over time and with different social attitudes as well as scientific discoveries about the origins and meanings of mental illness? What happens when we begin to think about mental illness as madness, as a malleable concept constantly shifting its meaning? We thus look at the meanings associated with "general paralysis of the insane" in the nineteenth century and autism today in regard to disability. In this case study we examine the claims by scholars such as the anthropologist Emily Martin and the psychiatrist Kay Jamison as to the relationship between mental illness, disability, and creativity. Today, the health sciences have become concerned with mental illness as a form of disability. How does this change the meaning of madness for practitioners and patients?

Madness?

With interest in mental illness from the standpoint of the growing field of disability studies comes a problem for the medical humanities.[1] Is it possible to discuss what may well be the most stigmatizing form of illness or disability in the West without understanding the complexity of the tradition in which it stands? The diagnostic history of mental illness is entangled with the history of madness as a social convention, a history that colors even the contemporary debates about the meanings and forms of mental illness in our age of brain imagery and neuroanatomy. These historical images shape the world of the medical professional as well as that of the layperson. We all carry conflicting and competing images of what mental illness means and how it is to be affectively as well as intellectually understood. Such images impact the meanings associated with the science of mental illness as well as the reception and self-perception of those who are disabled because of mental illness. There is no persistent distinction between images from the world of the health sciences dealing with mental illness/health and these popular images.[2] These images are interchangeable, each reifying the other. Mental illness is real because it fulfills our expectations of the image of madness; mental health is the alternative to such images. This is not to claim that mental health and mental illness do not exist—only that the boundaries between them are felt to be more rigid because of how we imagine madness. Indeed, the interpretability, flexibility, and malleability of the symptoms of mental illness (as with all symptoms of illness) over time reflect the expectations built on the interplay of popular and medical images.

It seems clear that mental illnesses, which allopathic medicine now defines as neurological rather than psychiatric, have different meanings attached to them in the past than in the present. For example general paralysis of the insane (G.P.I.), first diagnosed as a psychiatric category in 1822 by Antoine Bayle, was suggested to have a neurological cause as early as 1857 (by Friedrich von Esmnarch). In the latter half of the nineteenth century, this association between neurology and symptoms of madness was only whispered about. The double stigma concerning mental illness and sexually transmitted diseases meant that the possible relation between the two was rarely articulated. It was only after 1913, when Hideyo Noguchi and J. W. Moore were able to find syphilis spirochetes in virtually all of the sufferers, that G.P.I. was rebranded as tertiary neurosyphilis. But not all of the sufferers of G.P.I., with its clear and marked symptoms (frozen irregular pupils, diminished Babinski reflex, radical shifts in mental states, including depression and memory loss leading to dementia), turned out to have syphilis. Some were simply mad, as all with G.P.I. had been before 1913.[3]

The image of the person with G.P.I. is to be found in the early twentieth century as the "mad man" without any reference to the putative cause of the illness. Thus Clifford Beers, the founder of the National Committee for Mental Hygiene, (one of the very first disability advocacy groups in 1909) recounts in his autobiography *A Mind that Found Itself* (1908) seeing:

> another victim, forty-five years of age, was one who had formerly been a successful man of affairs. His was a forceful personality, and the traits of his sane days influenced his conduct when he broke down mentally. He was in the expansive phase of paresis, a phase distinguished by an exaggerated sense of well-being, and by delusions of grandeur which are symptoms of this form as well as of several other forms of mental disease. Paresis, as everyone knows, is considered incurable and victims of it seldom live more than three or four years. In this

> instance, instead of trying to make the patient's last days comfortable, the attendants subjected him to a course of treatment severe enough to have sent even a sound man to an early grave. I endured privations and severe abuse for one month at the State Hospital. This man suffered in all ways worse treatment for many months.[4]

This image of the oppressed insane is a commonplace in the world of disability advocacy. It is the image of the mad, not the bad, of the disordered, not the infected.

Hidden in the background of paresis even before the discovery of its actual etiology was the assumption of sexual license. Thus in the same year that Beers published his account, Elisabeth Förster-Nietzsche successfully brought suit to defend the memory of her brother, the philosopher Friedrich Nietzsche, who had died in 1900 after a complete mental collapse a dozen years earlier. The biographer of Nietzsche's friend Franz Overbeck mentioned in his account that Nietzsche may have died of G.P.I. The stigma of a sexually transmitted disease, even hinted at, was enough for the court to support her charges of libel, and the offending pages were removed from the volume.[5] Yet one of the themes that contributed to Overbeck's claim connecting Nietzsche's illness to infection was the view, very prevalent in the literature of the time, that such madness was one of the sources of true genius.[6] We can see how malleable such a retrospective etiology—and its implications—might be in the more recent retrospective diagnosis of Nietzsche's final illness as bipolar disorder. Unlike G.P.I., bipolar disorder is a disease without moral overtones because it does not invoke the same suspicion of sexual license. A diagnosis of bipolar disorder does, however, carry with it the assumption of some type of genetic cause, something that also would not have pleased Nietzsche's sister.[7]

Bipolar Disorder

The anthropologist Emily Martin sees herself as "mad"—she uses this term in the preface to her book to provide a context for her account of bipolar disorder/manic depression in the United States today.[8] Clinically diagnosed as bipolar, she repeatedly documents the symptoms of her illness. She has hallucinations including that of the "sinister figure, a cold gray gargoyle, perched tenaciously on [her] shoulder, looking at what [she] was writing . . . and muttering a devastatingly negative commentary" who haunted the very act of her writing.[9] What that "cold gray gargoyle" is reading over her shoulder is indeed her study of "mania . . . a new continent with a distant frontier, whose receding horizon invites exploration and development."[10] Actually, she uses this geographical phrase to describe the pharmaceutical companies seeking new drugs and new markets—but it is a very accurate view of Martin's mapping of modern manic depression in the age of psychopharmacology.

The question of madness as a disability invites a paradox: Can you be simultaneously "mad" and "rational," a "sufferer" and an "observer"? Certainly modern anthropology has wrestled with the problem of being both observer and participant, but what if the observer is mad? Martin sets this dichotomy at the core of her understanding of bipolar illness. Is mental illness ("madness") really incompatible with rational or (perhaps less stigmatizing) productive behavior? She is certainly not the first mad person to ask this question.

At the very beginning of the twentieth century Daniel Paul Schreber (1842–1911), lawyer, jurist, and failed parliamentary candidate, wrote and then published a book-length account of his mental illness.[11] The text first appeared in 1903, and he and it were later the prized subjects of studies by Sigmund Freud in his "Psycho-analytic notes on an autobiographical account of a case of paranoia (*dementia paranoids*)" (1910). Freud's interest was spurred on by C. G. Jung's advocacy of the text. The text was also of interest to the Nobel Prize winner Elias Canetti,[12] the psychoanalyst Jacques Lacan,[13] and the Marxists Gilles Deleuze and Félix Guattari.[14] Schreber published his account to prove to the director of the Dresden asylum in which he was hospitalized that he was not mad. He argued that mad people, even crazy lawyers, simply couldn't write books. He wrote his book, won his case, and was released (only to relapse and be rehospitalized decades later). The interest in his case as an example of psychopathology by the wide range of thinkers mentioned above was spurred by the very text that provided egress for him from the asylum.

The claim that certain abilities provide proof of sanity is not unique to Schreber and his authorship. A similar line of thinking can be seen in the series of events that led the brilliant art historian Aby Warburg to be released from his involuntary hospitalization in Ludwig Binswanger's sanatorium in Kreuzlingen from 1921 to 1924. He was diagnosed as "incurably schizoid," driven by paranoid fantasies of danger to himself and his family. There he held a talk on his "Reminiscences from a Journey to the Pueblo Indians," later posthumously published as "A Lecture on the Serpent Ritual." Warburg had seen this ritual on his visit to the Pueblos of northern New Mexico between December 1895 and May 1896. His presentation convinced Binswanger that he could now be released as "normal."[15]

Emily Martin reads the paradox between the rational and the insane as the key to understanding the very nature of bipolar disorder and its new function in American (and one can extrapolate—global) society. The commonplace that Schreber or Warburg successfully countered was that the mind of the "mentally ill" is inherently fragmented and incoherent. Mental health meant the unity of all parts of the psyche, proven, for instance, by the writing of books. Mental illness signaled the disruption of such unity. No internal multiplicity of the sense of the self could exist in healthy people. In the nineteenth century, the insane could regain their coherence and their reason through orderly living—moral treatment—and thus recover their sense of full personhood.[16] Asylums mirrored the institutions of society, holding dances for the inmates, providing work, mimicking an imagined ordered life into which the mad would eventually return to sanity and to society. This was the classic claim of the reformed asylum of the nineteenth century in which social structures, such as weekly dances, were seen as therapeutic as they both mimicked the sane world beyond the asylum and helped patients prepare to be reintegrated into that world. Living with mental illness meant being insane. It meant accepting the role of the mad person in the society, beyond order and redemption.

The individuals whom Martin meets in the 1990s in bipolar support groups live with their bipolar disorder even when they manage it with drugs. Her account shows that individuals diagnosed as bipolar are quite aware of their multiple aspects and the course of their illness. In fact, these individuals try, often with some success, to manage the radical alternation of their moods from highs to lows without losing their sense of disorder—the lived experience of all of the states of bipolar disorder encompassing the highs and the lows as well as a drug-provided alternative. The individuals she observes manage their lives, whether successfully or unsuccessfully, taking into account the knowledge that their chronic mental illness is part of who they are and will always be.

Madness and Creativity

Yet Martin's argument goes beyond just seeing how medicated bipolar individuals deal with their illness: she argues that at least one aspect of bipolar disorder is today seen as a model for a certain type of "healthy" or at least productive behavior in society. This positive reading of the manic comes to be part of the way that bipolar individuals internalize their illness. The "manic" aspect of their illness has come to be praised in the modern world as a positive character quality rather than as a sign of illness. According to Martin's insightful tabulation, corporate leaders such as Steve Jobs (of Apple) or Richard Branson (of Virgin) are seen as manic because they are risk-takers. Being manic in this sense is one of our definitions of success. Taking risks, acting beyond the limits of social boundaries, demanding the right to alter the world—all are signs of the successful entrepreneur as well as the manic patient.

Indeed, Martin shows how self-labeled manic-depressives—such as the Johns Hopkins psychologist Kay Jamison, the 1990s poster girl for bipolar disorder—create genealogies of successful "bipolar" people. Drawing on famous individuals from Edgar Allan Poe to Vincent van Gogh to Virginia Woolf and Jackson Pollack and Theodore Roosevelt and beyond, these genealogies are engineered to show that true creativity is in no way pathological, that being bipolar is simply another form of being creative.[17] Indeed, bipolar disorder traced through these genealogies emerges as the most valued source for all true creativity. Jamison thus quietly inserts herself and her book in this genealogy, making more or less the same claim as Schreber or Warburg. Such a claim that inexorably links creativity and madness is seen by Jamison and other such commentators as being ancient (and therefore universal), having its first articulation in Plato's theory of the "furores." Though Plato clearly distinguishes between creative madness and mental illness, Renaissance writers such as Marsilio Ficino elides these into the commonplace that madness is creativity. As Rudolph and Margot Wittkower note,

> Seneca's often quoted dictum: "*nullum magnum ingenium sine mixtura dementiae fuit*"—"there never has been great talent without some touch of madness"—would seem to express this point of view. In actual fact, Seneca's further comment leaves no doubt that he referred to the Platonic fire of divine inspiration rather than to insanity.[18]

By the nineteenth century, the view that madness and creativity were inexorably linked had become a commonplace within clinical psychiatry, especially in the work of Cesare Lombroso (1836–1909) and Paul Moebius (1853–1907). This claim, fostered by disability advocates for the mentally ill, more often than not collides with the lived experience of people with bipolar disorder whose mania is as destructive to their lives as is their depression. This lived experience stands in sharp contrast to a contemporary culture that claims the manic state as a truly productive one.

Now this, too, is a paradox that Martin avoids: she understands very well that the label manic is not the same as the lived experience of people with bipolar disorder, that creativity can be destroyed by the illness as well as furthered by it, that an individual such as Kay Jamison merely being able to write her brilliant and well-received book, is not a proof of the positive nature of the experience of illness for all those who live with it.[19] Indeed, Jamison's accomplishment is not even proof of the value of mania as a wellspring to creativity. It is quite possible to write in spite of and not because of one's illness—which is an answer to those who claim that creativity is proof of the value of mental illness.

Martin shows how the claims of a special creative potential in people with bipolar disorder collide with the life experience of manic-depressive individuals. For Martin sees that the changing categories of mental illness reflect societal images of what madness is and that those who are diagnosed as mentally ill shape their perception of their illness based on these changing expectations. "Does society claim that I am creative because I am bipolar?—then I had better live out that claim." As Martin notes, when you are given a diagnosis, that diagnosis becomes part of who you are.[20] She does not claim that madness is merely an invention of society. She is quite happy to speak of the biological and perhaps even genetic underpinnings of bipolar illness. But she sees that the lived experience of mental illness is altered by the changing meanings ascribed to it. Thus in the nineteenth century mania was seen as a feminine quality (enthusiasm) unhealthily present in men, while depression was a masculine quality (seriousness) present in women. Today, the claims are quite reversed, and mania has become the sign of a successful male competitor such as Branson or Jobs.

The view that diagnostic categories reflect social meaning and impact on the individual's sense of themselves is certainly not only true of mental illness. Some people with cancer (an unspoken word a generation ago) now proudly wear a pink ribbon. Breast cancer has become socially acceptable as *the* woman's illness, even though many more women die today of heart disease than breast cancer. The still unspeakable disease of men is prostate cancer. It is an illness that impacts many more men than the numbers of women who suffer from breast cancer and evokes the same type of sexual mutilation now answered by the pink ribbon. There is a little-known blue ribbon movement for prostate cancer (pink for girls; blue for boys). But few wear these ribbons today. The meanings as well as the rituals that are attributed to suffering from a disease shift as we rethink their function in society. Images of healthy and ill are formed and focused by societal pressures to create concrete ideas of illness. As Edward Bernays, one of the creators of modern advertising, wrote about public images, "any person or organization depends ultimately on public approval, and is therefore faced with the problem of engineering the public's consent to a program or goal."[21] This is equally true of the meanings associated with representations of mental illness.

One of Martin's claims is that evidence-based medicine creates clearly differentiated and self-limited categories of mental illness. These categories are often defined by the responses to drugs provided by the pharmaceutical companies who need to identify patient populations they can cure. Such claims not only define the very nature of the disease but also the individual's response. "I am bipolar" is a very different claim than "I have debilitating periods of depression and mania." Martin is in no way anti-pharmacology. She documents her own use of (and benefit from) psychotropic drugs. Yet she shows how drugs are given personalities by the drug companies (in their ads to physicians and in the public media) and by patients alike. Zoloft is, according to one user, "like a little robin's egg, it has that blue color and it represents hope."[22] (A very different blue from that of the prostate cancer ribbon!) If "I am bipolar," this is the perfect drug to answer my sense of hopelessness. The shape, color, and form of drugs, as Martin carefully documents in her field work in the drug companies, are very purposefully worked out: red is a bad color, as it seems to evoke the hectic intensity of mania rather than counter it; blue is claimed to be a calming and peaceful color. All are part of a culture of defining mental illness and its treatment, which shifts from social group to social group and epoch to epoch. What disables the individual with mental illness may not only be the illness they have but the meanings they and their world attach to that illness. Are they disabled when they write about their mental states, and, if so, what does disability mean in this context?

Madness and Disability

It is evident that to attempt to capture the relationship between madness and disability is to define one ambiguous and constantly shifting term by another. Madness has for centuries had legal and medical meanings; those meanings are more tangled and subject to political/ideological pressures than ever today in light of the framing of madness as a type of disability. For madness has now not only to figure itself in relation to ideas about competency, moral ability, curability, etc., but also in relation to questions of access, stigma, and advocacy.[23] Madness thus evokes not only a wide range of stereotypes of psychological difference (from the Greeks to the present), but also the lived experience of those who understand themselves and are understood as being mad. The term suggests the medical, social, and cultural categories dealing with all forms of psychic pain that came under the purview of alienists, psychiatrists, and neurologists. By contrast, madness can also be understood from a patient/client/inmate perspective rather than that of a psychiatric practitioner or clinician's perspective.

What seems to define madness in relationship to disability is the concept of psychic pain (or anguish or suffering). This certainly plays a major role in Emily Martin's account of bipolar disorder. The very existence of psychic pain, for example, is today thought to be a contested source of knowledge, having its modern origins in John Locke's view that "Pain [is] . . . sometimes occasioned by disorder in the Body, sometimes by Thoughts of the Mind."[24] However else madness has been defined, such psychic pain was and remains a litmus test for madness, whether as a reason for intervention or as a perceived source for greater insight into the mad and their creative capacities.

A broad understanding of madness therefore must account for medical perspectives (both allopathic and complementary/alternative practices) as well as multiple social, political, and cultural understandings of madness and mad people, all fluid and ever moving across the world. Every society has its own categories and perspectives and experiences of madness—from melancholia in ancient Athens to spirit madness in modern Evangelical churches; from the representations of madness of American medical missionaries in China in the nineteenth century to those selling cures for madness in the botanicas of the Dominicans in New York City today. Across the globe, societies see categories of madness as something that impinge on human activity, for ill or for good, and with a variety of meanings that generate a variety of interpretations. The realities of what constitutes madness in any given society or community or historical moment are constantly shifting: symptoms change and their meanings seem always in flux. Even as different etiologies and meanings of madness emerge to explain the somatic, psychological, social, and cultural causes of madness, psychic pain remains central to all of these categories. Madness may be the antithesis of what is called normal. Likewise, it may be related to other categories of illness and pain, or be a state that transcends the normal.[25] Similarly, if we explore madness not in the realm of a medicalized society but in the parallel world of the law, then madness takes on yet other colorations. The two realms are intertwined. From the forensic definitions of madness created by the Romans, which focused on competency, aging, and property, to the McNaughton rule of Victorian England, which focused on the moral ability to know right for wrong in the case of Daniel McNaughton, who attempted to assassinate the British Prime Minister Robert Peel in 1843, we see legal definitions of madness that parallel and mimic medical and social definitions of madness. But these legal definitions are also autonomous. Today, one does not speak of madness but rather of psychiatric illness/diagnosis in the world of law. Yet the contemporary functional definition within the law remains inherently one developed by Victorian alienists. This often leads to a complicated political response to the use of the incompetency defense in court, especially in high-profile cases of political assassination (such as in the murder of President James Garfield by Charles Guiteau in 1881) or infanticide (the use of the postnatal psychosis in the case of Susan Smith in 1995). In both cases the defense, using a version of the McNaughton rule, was unsuccessful. At least a few American states (Montana, Idaho, and Utah) have now banned this defense.[26]

It is thus imperative to sort out what we mean when we use the categories of madness and psychic pain that define our object. Once we have settled on a particular definition/construct of madness, then we can ask how these limits impact on our understanding of those who are defined by these limits. Central to all definitions of madness is the idea of innate difference that is associated with it. This stereotype may be positive—debates about creativity and madness, for instance, go back to the ancients—but most have negative consequences. These include physically isolating the mad from society, refusing to give the same rights to the mad as to other citizens, and seeing madness as a diminution of one's humanity.

Toward a History of Madness

The Greeks regarded madness as the result of a physical imbalance of the four humors (black bile, yellow bile, phlegm, and blood), the bodily fluids that they believed regulated health and temperament (thus they created melancholic, choleric, phlegmatic, and sanguine temperaments and their attendant illnesses). The Chinese at the same time conceived of madness as an imbalance of the primal forces of yin and yang. Jewish beliefs, mirrored in the accounts in the *Tanach* (Old Testament), stressed moral failing and divine intervention as a primary cause of madness as in the case of Nebuchadnezzar (Daniel 1 4:31–33) but also as in Samuel 10:6 the voice of the often unrecognized prophet. All of these cultures placed the mad in a separate category: for some a higher one of prophecy and illumination, but for most one of marginality and exclusion. All developed some types of therapeutic interventions for the latter, not necessarily for the former.

Roman and, later, medieval medicine and society made the distinction between the naturally born idiot and the lunatic, terms that overlap with and permeate medieval law and medicine. The former were not seen as treatable, but the latter were. The moral stigma and legal treatment of both, however, were clearly parallel. The question of causation mixed theological, physiological, and mystical etiologies, to varying degrees at different times and places. The means of treatment were similarly mixed: from spiritual exorcism to the use of somatic interventions such as diet to restore mental balance and physical control and restrain individuals from actions that could harm their estates. This was also the case in Islamic medicine, which had transmitted much of Greco-Roman social and medical attitudes on madness in the Middle Ages to Europe but which also was permeated by Christian and Jewish medical practice in Europe and beyond. Thus Sura 4:5 of the Qur'an: "Give not unto the foolish what is in your keeping of their wealth, which Allah hath given you to maintain; but feed and clothe them from it, and speak kindly unto them." This is a cultural translation of the Roman medico-forensic notions of "furiosus" and "non compos mentis" in limiting economic damage to an estate by a mad parent's fiscal irresponsibility, a notion that is itself linked to the theological understanding of madness from the New Testament (Matthew 4:24).[27]

As the notion of the hospital evolved in the early Middle Ages, specialized institutions for the mad developed as early as AD 705 in Baghdad. This tradition had spread into Western Europe by the late Middle Ages in Spain and Western Europe. While a form of medical incarceration appeared for diseases such as leprosy and madness, the mad were rarely permanently housed in such facilities. Unlike lepers, who were understood to be contagious, they were usually incarcerated for a limited time, usually because of the costs to local communities for extended confinement, and then released. Leprosy and madness generated a sense of dread derived from the prevalent images of the leper and the insane. It was of little surprise that specific institutions grew up to socially isolate these sources of public anxiety. By the Renaissance, madness also became a conceit for the view that one's mad actions could be a sign of sanity in a world gone mad. As William Shakespeare has Hamlet say (1601): "I essentially am not in madnesse, But mad in craft." (iii. iv. 171). This view of madness as a metaphor for sanity in an unstable world would become a commonplace of Romantic views of insanity and, indeed, part of the idea of madness thereafter.

By the nineteenth century in Western Europe the idea of a moral treatment of the insane as well as the isolation of the idiots seen as inherently incurable from the treatable lunatics was generally accepted. Moral treatment aimed at the return of the lunatics to their proper place in the world through the moral and secular correction of the misunderstandings of the world and their inappropriate actions. Thus the practice, mentioned above, of weekly dances for the inmates to reestablish the moral order of their inmates. Led by lay directors, such clinical facilities gave way in the course of the nineteenth century to an ever-greater degree of medicalization across Europe and North America, so much so that their directors by the close of the century were virtually all medically trained alienists. This development in treatment paralleled the professionalization of psychiatry and neurology and the creation of a systematic set of diagnostic categories as well as treatments. Most of these were based on physiological principles, though strongly psychological interventions paralleled them at the close of the century. Suddenly madness as a category gave way to other terms such as "affective disorder," as J. C. Bucknill and D. H. Tuke state in their standard *Manual of Psychological Medicine*.[28]

Even so, the nineteenth century placed its emphasis on somatic definitions of madness. Wilhelm Griesinger in 1868 writes: "The so-called mental illnesses are found in individuals suffering from brain- and nerve illness."[29] By the 1890s, this view seems to be universal in Western psychiatry. The neurologists of the time, such as the young Sigmund Freud, assume this as a fact but question the relationship between organic sources of madness and the wide range of psychological manifestations of mental illness. Freud begins a movement, psychoanalysis, that accounts for the widest range of mental states as potentially leading to psychic pain yet without any direct organic cause. Indeed, Freud's great insight is that bodily symptoms, such as paralysis, can have purely psychological causes and should be treated by psychological interventions such as talk therapy rather than physical treatments such as electrotherapy.[30]

The somatization of madness increased across the twentieth century, but it came at a cost. More and more symptoms were related to specific neurological deficits such as dementia. Developmental disorders came to be sorted out from illnesses with complex neurological causes—reductively dividing environmental diseases from genetic ones, for example—and thus further separating out those diseases seen as purely illness of the spirit, the psyche, or the mind. Thus the idiot and the lunatic, often housed in the same state institution through the nineteenth century, were by the early twentieth century seen as manifesting quite different social and medical causes.[31] Indeed biological interventions such as sterilization dealt with such individuals not to aid them but to improve society by eliminating their ability to reproduce. As the United States Supreme Court justice Oliver Wendell Holmes, Jr. concluded in affirming the Commonwealth of Virginia's eugenic sterilization law:

> It is better for all the world, if instead of waiting to execute degenerate offspring for crime, or to let them starve for their imbecility, society can prevent those who are manifestly unfit from continuing their kind. The principle that sustains compulsory vaccination is broad enough to cover cutting the Fallopian tubes. Three generations of imbeciles are enough.[32]

Biological definitions of madness generated a wide range of biological interventions to limit and control madness.

Yet the greater the detailed knowledge of the causes and meanings of madness the more the boundaries that defined it begin to shift. Thus general paralysis of the insane, the most common diagnosis for psychiatric patients in the nineteenth-century asylum, came to be recognized as the last stages of syphilitic infection following the development of a specific test for the syphilis spirochetes in 1906; it thus became a potentially treatable neurological disease rather than a form of mental illness. After specific treatments for syphilis were developed, "general paralysis of the insane" simply vanished from the diagnostic repertoire of most physicians who dealt with madness, and the treatment of its characteristic symptoms entered other medical specialties.

The desire in the twentieth century was to find more and more cases in which madness was the result of specific biological, neurological, or genetic factors. Eugenic interventions, such as sterilization, came to be repudiated (if slowly) after the horrors of the Holocaust and its eugenically inspired mass murder of "inferior races" as well as the disabled. Compulsory sterilization laws for madness existed in the United States from 1897 to well into the late 1970s, and sterilization still occurs in isolated cases, such as the California prison system, until today. In light of the Holocaust, post–WWII medicine sought specific biomedical interventions (mainly psychotropic drugs) that could have an impact on the symptoms of madness, then defined in terms of psychosis (a lesser or greater loss of the psychic connection to reality) and neurosis (the impairment of rationality that leads to psychic pain).[33]

Developmental disorders seem to have been bracketed in the search for a cure for a drug to cure madness. Yet the discovery of DNA in 1952 and the subsequent discovery of the specific mutations for Down's syndrome in 1959 were more or less simultaneous with the first uses of lithium to treat the symptoms of depression and Thorazine (chlorpromazine hydrochloride) in 1950 to treat the symptoms of schizophrenia. The idea that there could be a genetic intervention to prevent all such developmental disorders is also an artifact of this post–WWII science as much as the now seemingly universal use of psychotropic drugs, from that first antipsychotic medication in the 1950s to mood enhancers (Prozac) to drugs to treat hyperactivity (Ritalin). The expansion of drug treatment was first heralded by patients and physicians alike as effective interventions but quickly became a target of patient and social discontent given massive side effects as well as the over-prescription of many such drugs to ever-widening categories of individuals. Madness seemed to become quotidian, and yet the stigma of madness remained.

With the expansion of psychotropic drug use, the patient self-consciously became the client and with such shift of definition became more and more self-aware. Twentieth- and twenty-first-century patient populations are now, in effect, consumers of medical care, and as consumers they organize and make demands—demands that range from the call for de-institutionalization and the closing of large public facilities housing individuals believed to be unable to function in the world to the desire to be released from the negative stigma of madness.

The rise of a contested science of madness in the nineteenth century provides a basis for the medical treatment of mental states as illnesses in the systematic classification of forms of mental (and other) illness. Begun in 1893 by Jacques Bertillon as a positivistic description of illness based on observable symptoms and analogous to his work in criminology, this soon became a global phenomenon. Though it was revised in 1898 by the American Public Health Association as the *International Statistical Classification of Diseases, Injuries and Causes of Death* (ICD), it was only after 1948 that the World Health Organization's *International Statistical Classification of Diseases and Related Health Problems* appeared. It became the gold standard for international psychiatric classification, especially after its eighth edition of 1968. In 1973, the *Diagnostic and Statistical Manual of the American Psychiatric Association*, which had first appeared in 1952, assumed a global role in unifying the terminology for psychiatric classification. What was remarkable about these widely accepted means of describing mental illness is that they codified the contemporary views and attitudes toward madness globally rather than locally. And by doing so they claimed a scientific uniformity that existed only within their own closed systems.

In the 1960s, alternative perspectives on madness began to emerge in the works of Erving Goffman, R. D. Laing, and Thomas Szasz, offering a re-examination of the social causes of madness. These had a powerful impact on the de-medicalization of madness among feminists and gay activists in the 1970s. Where Goffman saw the asylum as a repressive means of social control, Szasz saw madness as invented by the patient as well as society. Laing saw madness as the "healthy' product of sick social or familial structures. All of these models contributed to the growing patient empowerment movement of the time and began to shape the idea of disability beyond the medical model of rehabilitation (taken from interventions related to deafness and blindness) that had dominated the field from the eighteenth century.[34] The idea of a relativization of madness (now freed of any medical implication) first appeared in sociological work in France in the work of Georges Canguilhem in the 1940s and, later, with his student Michel Foucault in the 1960s. In *Folie et Déraison. Histoire de la folie à l'âge Classique* (1961), Foucault dismissed the antithesis of sanity and madness as the result of medical power.[35] One concrete result was that entire categories of madness such as homosexuality (in 1973) and premenstrual syndrome (in 1987) came to be dismissed from psychiatric diagnosis. More generally, the very idea of madness came to be suspect as stigmatizing rather than diagnosing.

Disability

Medical discourses of rehabilitation and disability inspired the creation of the category of psychiatric disability following the 1980 World Health Organization's *International Classification of Impairments, Disabilities and Handicaps'* definition of disability as the *result* of illness. Thus a psychiatric disability can be the result of a psychiatric impairment, which can be the source of the stigma of madness that impinges on the ability of the individual to function in the community. Different from other disabilities, such as developmental disabilities, psychiatric disabilities are seen as episodic and intermittent. But here the acknowledgement of the causality of the stigma of madness does not touch the underlying medical assumptions about the meaning of madness.

One reaction to this medicalized model of disability within the disability rights movement (and its allied academic field of disability studies) is to begin to see all forms of mental ability and emotional stability as ranged on a spectrum. The concept of a spectrum of human psychological/mental diversity comes as an answer to the older model of psychiatric disability. Harvey Blume coined the term "neurodiversity" in 1998 as a defining quality of being human: "Neurodiversity may be every bit as crucial for the human race as biodiversity is for life in general. Who can say what form of wiring will prove best at any given moment? Cybernetics and computer culture, for example, may favor a somewhat autistic cast of mind."[36] This followed from work in disability studies that spoke of the "extraordinary" body, the "rejected" body, the "recovering" body, or, more recently, the "problem" body.[37] Disability thus dealt with the "reception or construction of [the] difference" presented by a "physical or mental impairment."[38] Here one suddenly has the idea of the extraordinary, rejected, recovering, or problem mind.

Such ideas of madness and disability develop parallel to the growth of popular interest in autism, which also comes to be the litmus test of the new test case for madness within disability studies. As Paul Heilker and Melanie Yergeau note, "Public awareness and public discourse about autism are approaching critical mass."[39] Medically, autism has been defined as a psychiatric category since the mid twentieth century. It is now seen as a developmental disorder with genetic or environmental causes. Certainly the flawed claims about MMR vaccination as the cause of autism colored its reevaluation at the end of the twentieth century by stressing the potential elimination of autism through social action rather that through genetic or medical intervention.

Today, autism is increasingly seen as an alternative, even a preferred mental state, rather than as a deficit. It is the answer to Erich Fromm's view that madness in modern society is a sign of humanity's fall from "biophilia"—that is, from a sense of relatedness, rootedness, and orientation.[40] Autism has come to be a sign that individual autonomy can challenge and often overcome notions of social isolation.[41] The fascination with idiot savants in the late-twentieth-century public sphere (such as the autistic Raymond in Barry Levinson's film *Rain Man* [1988]) gives way to a new focus on the autistic individual as a representative of neurodiversity. Asperger's Syndrome is the new norm.[42]

This framing of autism draws on debates about the autonomy of the client/patient from the 1960s and the image of a broader spectrum of mental health held by disability studies scholars. It rejects any sense of the autist as being severely impaired and in need of special facilities, instead considering him only differently enabled. Indeed, both activists and scholars of disability have promoted the growing sense that autists are actually better enabled in a world that does not recognize their abilities. This is the theme of the bestselling 2003 novel by Mark Haddon, *The Curious Incident of the Dog in the Night-Time.* (See the various positions in the special issue of the *Disability Studies Quarterly* on neurodiversity devoted to autism.)[43] This view is very much in line with the reinterpretation of bipolar disorder as the source of creativity by bipolar writers such as Jamison.

The need for public facilities for severely impacted autistic people has diminished as quickly in the twenty-first century as it did for the mad in general during the 1960s. The source of this decline is the sense that autistic individuals must function as part of a newly redefined public sphere that, according to law and custom, is now open to them, no matter how severe their individual state. The model for this is the treatment of Asperger's syndrome rather than severe, debilitating autism. Thus the politics of disability and madness can be clearly seen in the debates about autism in the twenty-first century. The Americans with Disabilities Act (1990) defines disabling madness as "any mental or psychological disorder, such as mental retardation, organic brain syndrome, emotional or mental illness, and specific learning disabilities" that "substantially limits one or more major life activities of an individual" or that cause one to be "regarded as having such an impairment." Both aspects of this definition assume a psychiatric diagnosis. The British Disability Discrimination Act (1995) follows the standard handbooks of psychiatric diagnosis as well as the idea that such forms of mental illness must be chronic or recurrent.

In 2011, the Neurodevelopmental Work Group, led by Susan Swedo, MD, senior investigator at the National Institute of Mental Health, was tasked with revising the category of autism in the standard American diagnostic handbook of psychiatry, the *Diagnostic and Statistical Manual of Mental Disorders, fifth edition* (DSM-5). They first suggested that the definitions of autism spectrum disorder be reworked and simplified. In DSM-IV, patients could be diagnosed with four separate disorders: autistic disorder, Asperger's disorder, childhood disintegrative disorder, or the catchall diagnosis of pervasive developmental disorder not otherwise specified. It was proposed to unify and clarify these categories.

The reaction from the autism community in 2011, now well organized into political lobbying organizations with substantial funding raising capacity and celebrity spokespeople, was swift and damning, seeing this medical decision as impacting on the funding for autistic clients as well as the exclusion of certain forms of autism from coverage in the law. The claim was that Asperger's syndrome and about 25 percent of those with other diagnoses of autism would not qualify under the new DSM-5 category. The psychiatrists who suggested the reforms to DSM-5 quickly backtracked and the revision of the diagnostic category of autism spectrum disorders was again revised. When DSM-5 was eventually published in 2013, it reflected the political interaction between disability advocacy groups and the psychiatric community.[44]

The autists who successfully pressured the drafting committee for DSM-5 acted in complex ways. They demanded more medicalization (or at least reversing a trend toward de-medicalization) but at the same time they were able to exhibit their political clout as an interest group. Since the drift of most disability activism is to de-medicalize disability, this is a counterthrust. Neurodiversity is their cry, but they also want to preserve their medical coverage and legal protections. The medical model for madness is still potent even as the disability world begins to try and erode its power. The autists *do* erode the power of the medical community by putting pressure on them to reverse their decision, but the result is more rather than less medicalization. For autists as well as others diagnosed with mental illness or neurological disorder today, adopting the medical model of madness can still confer tactical advantage for some disability groups. Emily Martin showed this in the case of bipolar disorder, but it may well now be a truism in terms of how contemporary society deals with madness.

Notes

1. Paul K. Longmore and Lauri Umansky, eds., *The New Disability History: American Perspectives* (New York: New York University Press, 2001); Felicity Callard et al., *Mental Illness, Discrimination and the Law: Fighting for Social Justice* (New York: Wiley-Blackwell, 2012).
2. Ato Quayson, *Aesthetic Nervousness: Disability and the Crisis of Representation* (New York: Columbia University Press, 2007).
3. Claude Quétel, *History of Syphilis*, trans. J Braddock and B Pike (Cambridge: Polity Press, 1992).
4. Clifford Wittingham Beers, *A Mind that Found Itself*, 2nd ed. (New York: Longman, Green, 1910), 171.

5. Carl Albrecht Bernoulli, *Franz Overbeck und Friedrich Nietzsche, eine Freundschaft*, 2 vols. (Jena: Diederichs, 1908); Sander L. Gilman, *Begegnungen mit Nietzsche* (Bonn: Bouvier, 1981), XI–XIII.
6. Deborah Hayden, *Pox: Genius, Madness, and the Mysteries of Syphilis* (New York: Basic Books, 2003).
7. E. M. Cybulska, "The madness of Nietzsche: a misdiagnosis of the millennium?" *Hospital Medicine* 61, no. 8 (2000): 571–75.
8. Emily Martin, *Bipolar Expeditions: Mania and Depression in American Culture* (Princeton: Princeton University Press, 2007).
9. Ibid., xv.
10. Ibid., 15.
11. Daniel Paul Schreber, *Memoirs of My Nervous Illness*, trans. Ida Macalpine and Richard A Hunter (1903; repr., Cambridge, MA: Harvard University Press, 1988).
12. Elias Canetti, *Crowds and Power*, trans. Carol Stewart (1960; repr., New York: Farrar, Straus, and Giroux).
13. Jacques Lacan, *The Seminar of Jacques Lacan III: The Psychoses*, 1955–56 (New York: Routledge, 1992); he also discusses the text in one of his *écrits*, "On a Question prior to Any Possible Treatment of Psychosis" in 1958. This is available, among other translations, in Chapter Six of *Écrits: A Selection*, trans. Alan Sheridan (New York: Routledge, 1977).
14. Giles Deleuze and Felix Guattari, Anti-Oedipus, Capitalism and Schizophrenia, trans. Robert Hurley (1972; repr., New York: Penguin: 2009).
15. Aby Warburg, *Images from the Region of the Pueblo Indians of North America*, trans. Michael P. Steinberg (Ithaca: Cornell University Press, 1995); Davide Stimilli, ed., *Die unendliche Heilung. Aby Warburgs Krankengeschichte* (Berlin: Diaphanes Verlag, 2007).
16. Martin, 91.
17. Kay Redfield Jamison, *Touched with Fire: Manic-Depressive Illness and the Artistic Temperament* (New York: Free Press, 1996).
18. Rudolph Wittkower and Margot Wittkower, *Born Under Saturn: The Character and Conduct of Artists* (New York: Norton, 1969), 98.
19. Kay Redfield Jamison, *An Unquiet Mind: A Memoir of Moods and Madness* (New York: Knopf, 1995).
20. Martin, 129.
21. Edward Bernays, *Public Relations* (Norman: University of Oklahoma Press, 1952), 9.
22. Martin, 162.
23. Fred Pelka, *What We Have Done: An Oral History of the Disability Rights Movement* (Amherst, MA: University of Massachusetts Press, 2012).
24. John Locke, *Essay on Human Understanding* (1690) at http://www.ilt.columbia.edu/publications/Projects/digitexts/locke/understanding/chapter0220.html (accessed 22 September 2013). The passage referred to here appears in Book 2, chapter 20, on p. 113. Accessed May 2, 2012.
25. Sander L. Gilman, *Seeing the Insane: A Cultural History of Psychiatric Illustration* (New York: Wiley Interscience, 1982); Roy Porter, *Madness: A Brief History* (Oxford: Oxford University Press, 2003).
26. Candice Millard, *Destiny of the Republic: A Tale of Madness, Medicine and the Murder of a President* (New York: Doubleday, 2011); George

Rekers, *Susan Smith: Victim or Murderer* (Lakewood, CO: Glenbridge Publishing, 1995).

27. Daniel Robinson, *Wild Beasts and Idle Humors: The Insanity Defense from Antiquity to the Present* (Cambridge: Harvard University Press, 1998).
28. J. C. Bucknill and D. H. Tuke, *Manual of Psychological Medicine* (London: Blanchard and Lea, 1858), 125.
29. Wilhelm Griesinger, "Vorwort," *Archiv für Psychiatrie und Nervenkrankheiten* 1 (1868): iii–viii, here iii.
30. Sander L. Gilman, *The Case of Sigmund Freud: Medicine and Identity at the Fin de Siècle* (Baltimore: The Johns Hopkins University Press, 1993).
31. James W. Trent, Jr., *Inventing the Feeble Mind: A History of Mental Retardation in the United States* (Berkeley: University of California Press, 1994).
32. *Buck v. Bell* 274 (U.S. 200 1927)
33. Edward Shorter, *A History of Psychiatry: From the Era of the Asylum to the Age of Prozac* (New York: Wiley, 1998).
34. Henri-Jacques Stiker, *A History of Disability*, trans. William Sayers (Ann Arbor: University of Michigan Press, 1999).
35. Michel Foucault, *History of Madness*, ed. J. Khalfa, trans. J. Murphy (New York: Routledge, 2006).
36. Harvey Blume, "Neurodiversity," *The Atlantic*, September 30, 1998, http://www.theatlantic.com/doc/199809u/neurodiversity (accessed September 22, 2013).
37. They are, respectively: Rosemarie Garland-Thomson, *Extraordinary Bodies: Figuring Physical Disability in American Culture and Literature* (New York: Columbia University Press, 1997); Susan Wendell, *The Rejected Body: Feminist Philosophical Reflections on Disability* (New York: Routledge, 1996); G. Thomas Couser, *Recovering Bodies: Illness, Disability, and Lifewriting* (Madison: University of Wisconsin Press, 1997); Sally Chivers and Nicole Markotić, eds., *The Problem Body: Projecting Disability on Film* (Columbus: Ohio State University Press, 2010).
38. Lennard J. Davis, "Dr. Johnson, Amelia, and the Discourse of Disability in the 18th century," in *'Defects' Engendering the Modern Body, ed.* Helen Deutsch and Felicity Nussbaum (Ann Arbor: University Michigan Press, 2000), 54–74, here 56.
39. Paul Heilker and Melanie Yergeau, "Autism and Rhetoric," *College English* 73, no. 5 (2011): 485–497, here 485.
40. Erich Fromm, *The Sane Society* (New York: Henry Holt, 1955).
41. Stuart Murray, *Autism* (New York: Routledge, 2012).
42. Exemplified by the film *Temple Grandin*, directed by Mick Jackson, HBO Films, Ruby Films, 2010, a biopic that describes the youth of Temple Grandin, the iconic autist who is currently a professor at Colorado State University, and *Adam*, directed by Max Mayer, Olympus Pictures, Deer Path Productions, Northwood Productions, 2009, the account of a young man suffering from Asperger's syndrome.
43. Emily Thornton Savarese and Ralph James Savarese, eds., "Autism and the Concept of Neurodiversity," *Disability Studies Quarterly* 30 (2010): 1.
44. Allen Francis, *Saving Normal: An Insider's Revolt Against Out-of-Control Psychiatric Diagnosis, DSM-5, Big Pharma, and the Medicalization of Ordinary Life* (New York: William Morrow, 2013).

Questions

Is mental illness always a disability?

When can mental illness be understood as a positive rather than a negative state?

What does "creativity" mean, and how is it impacted by mental illness?

Who defines "mental illness"?

Is there a religious definition of mental illness?

Case Seven

Self-Harm and Mental Illness

Problems: Self-inflicted injury has a history. Part of understanding this history involves understanding how the meaning of self-harm as a symptom of mental illness changes over time. Do such changes undermine our assumptions about the need for continuity in diagnostic practice? Are surface symptoms simply malleable signs of an underlying disease process that is constant even as its cultural expression is varied? What does this paradox—the question of whether illness stays the same as culture changes or culture changes illness and the way in which this entanglement cannot be completely teased out—say about how ideas of madness are dependent on our understanding of who we are and how we relate to our bodies as well as to our psyches?

A Paradox?

Early in my career teaching at medical schools, I proposed a thought experiment to my students: "A patient comes to you with the following complaint. 'I am very unhappy with my left leg. I have always been unhappy with it. It causes me constant unhappiness. I wish to have it removed.' You examine the seemingly normal-appearing leg, ask about chronic pain, but are told only that it is the cause of constant unhappiness. You find neither somatic pathologies nor functional problems. What do you do?" The answer in the 1970s seemed crystal clear: refer the patient to a mental health specialist for further evaluation.

Yet had I given the class in the 1970s the same exercise about the patient's nose, the answer may well have been different. In a world of burgeoning cosmetic surgery for which a psychological rationale was both sufficient and necessary for undertaking an aesthetic procedure, the answer may well have been: "refer to a cosmetic surgeon." The rationale for an operation on a healthy (i.e., functioning) nose was provided in the 1890s by the Berlin surgeon Jacques Joseph and quickly made the standard for all cosmetic procedures, which were seen as surgery directed at curing the mind rather than repairing the body.[1]

The unhappy left leg could have been seen in the 1970s as a case of body integrity identity disorder (apotemnophilia), for which, at least in the 1990s, the surgical removal of healthy limbs was prophylactically undertaken. Specifically, this surgery occurred in Scotland with the aim of preventing self-mutilation as a symptom of mental illness.[2] Better, it was thought, to undertake the procedure medically than to risk a patient's death—the notion of undertaking to intervene in the underlying mental illness through nonsurgical means seemed not to be part of the argument.

Or, as Ilana Löwy shows in her *Preventative Strikes: Women, Precancer, and Prophylactic Surgery*, had the patient told me that her oncologist had discovered a "precancerous" familial pattern and suggested surgical intervention, my referral would have been to an oncological surgeon.[3] The rational for mastectomies to remove what might pose a risk for cancer comes about in the 1920s, well before our present means of prognosis using genetic information. (This information has now been coded by categories of "race," with Jewish women seen as a definable cohort at risk given the presence in some of them of the BRCA1 and 2 genetic mutations.) But the recent improvement in prognosis does not mean a clear rationale for the undertaking of such surgeries, any more than the use of psychological diagnosis is a litmus test for other such surgical interventions (as the debates about both apotemnophilia and cosmetic surgery show even today.) The underlying question is what constitutes the boundary between acceptable and unacceptable categories and how social factors impacts on clinical decision-making.

Self-Harm as a Moral Panic

In 2011 there is a sharp public awareness of self-harm across the world as a major issue of mental health.

> Cutting, burning, and other forms of deliberate self-harm are surprisingly common among adolescents. . . . Marjorie Wallace, chief executive of the English mental health charity SANE, told the BBC, "Our research shows that counter to common perception, people self-harm and continue to self-harm at times throughout their lives."[4]

In Singapore:

> experts . . . said they sensed a new trend of troubled teenage girls and even young women mutilating themselves in more "discreet" areas that are hidden by blouses and skirts. There may be several possible reasons, from mood disorders to self-esteem issues to peer pressure, as in a group initiation ritual.[5]

In India:

> cutting and self-mutilation are silent and often damaging cries for help, affecting roughly 25% of today's youth between the ages of 13 and 19. Most who self-injure are female but males do so as well. Whether suffering from depression, anxiety or another form of hurt or anger, self-injury is a painful yet private external expression of severe internal pain.[6]

While social service agencies and medical/psychiatric experts see this problem within their own models of understanding of mental health, this view of self-harm is widely accepted as a new social epidemic that religion, too, (using a medical model) has become engaged with it. In North Carolina, evangelical groups see this as a problem demanding intervention.

> Tami Lilly is the founder of Exodus Ministries, a nonprofit Christian mentoring program that helps people break the "generational patterns of abuse, poverty and addictions through the liberating knowledge of God's truths." . . . And Lilly is passionate about the need for such a ministry. "Some of the stories would shock you to hear what this generation is dealing with," she explains. "Kids are in so much pain that there is an epidemic of cutting and self-mutilation. Children as young as the third grade are attempting suicide!" Now she is on a mission to help end these cycles.[7]

Today this concern reflects a global moral panic about the inner lives of those now defined by "self-harming."

"Cutting and self-mutilation" is the focus of all of these popular reports. It has become the stuff of young adult fiction and graphic novels intended to provide models of how adolescents can deal with this new epidemic.[8] Yet in twenty-first-century popular culture there is a hierarchy of medical self-harm that stands in opposition to socially or medically acceptable "self-mutilation." The line is drawn between body modification and tattooing as well as even the most radical type of now acceptable medical practice such as preventative mastectomy and those categories of self-mutilation defined as symptoms of mental illness. The focus has been on "cutting," but the consensus is that the worse such self-mutilation is the rarer it is, particularly cases that escalate to self-amputation:

> Major SM refers to infrequent acts such as eye enucleation, castration, and limb amputation.

> Stereotypic SM refers to acts such as head banging and hitting, orifice digging, arm hitting, throat and eye gouging, self-biting, tooth extraction, and joint dislocation.
>
> Superficial/moderate SM refers to acts such as trichotillomania, nail biting, and skin picking and scratching, which comprise the compulsive type, and to skin cutting, carving, and burning, needle sticking, bone breaking, and interference with wound healing, which comprise the episodic and repetitive types.[9]

This litany of self-harm is cited from a paper by Armando R. Favazza, and we can use it to date the newest and now defining moment that brings "superficial/moderate" self-harm into contemporary popular and medical consciousness as a unique and major form of mental illness.

In 1987, Armando R. Favazza published *Bodies under Siege: Self-mutilation and Body Modification in Culture and Psychiatry.*[10] This work helped fix the notion of self-harm in the form of cutting in the public sphere, or—perhaps since the public sphere was ready for self-harm as a mass phenomenon—codified the "moral panic" around self-harm/self-mutilation. We shall see that self-harm and self-mutilation are actually overlapping but not identical categories. "Cutting" has become a new "moral panic" about the dangers confronting today's youth. A "moral panic" is an "episode, condition, person or group of persons" that have in recent times, been "defined as a threat to societal values and interests."[11] Thus Stanley Cohen in the early 1970s writes about the public reaction to the "mods and rockers" who haunted London streets during the 1960s. Self-harm is characterized, to continue to quote Cohen on other such manifestations, by "stylized and stereotypical" representation by the mass media, and a tendency for those "in power" (politicians, bishops, editors, and so on) to man the "moral barricades" and pronounce moral judgments. Moral panics need not be focused on "invented" categories such as witches; they can also be associated with real health problems in such a way as to magnify and shape their meanings. Individuals or groups relying on the assumptions underlying a "moral panic" can use "real" categories of illness to explain such health problems within the ideological focus of the time.

Today "cutting"—the new shorthand term and primary symptom in popular culture for self-harm—has become a moral panic. It thus occupies the same world of fear as eating disorders. As one commentator recently noted:

> There has been much gnashing of teeth in the media over our insatiable appetites, with blame being laid in diverse places: crisps, car culture, school vending machines, and oversized portions, which we apparently cannot resist. But if we start to look at obesity as part of a much bigger picture, more alarming and confusing ideas begin to emerge. We are not only seeing an unprecedented rise in levels of obesity, but also soaring rates of alcohol abuse, misuse of hard drugs, eating disorders, self-harm, and suicide. Stress and harm are highly contested definitions, but many people are living at a feverish pitch, which is erupting into all sorts of symptoms and propagating a booming market in self-help books. . . .[12]

The idea that "living at a feverish pitch" is the cause of specific instances of mental illnesses with specific sets of symptoms is a commonplace of nineteenth-century degeneration theory as promulgated by writers such as Max Nordau. But such moral panics do have moments of condensation, and these can be found in the late-twentieth-century focus on cutting no longer as a symptom but as a disease.

Favazza argues in the late twentieth century that self-mutilation is a universal cultural manifestation. He begins with an account of self-mutilation as rooted in cultural images from Tibetan tantric meditation and traces these images through to the creation of Franz Kafka's penal colony. He associates these examples not necessarily with self-mutilation as a form of mental illness but rather with practices of social mutilation, such as decapitation and scalping, or healing, or the adoration of relics of the saints.[13] Mutilation is "culturally and psychologically embedded in the profound, elemental experiences of healing, religion, and social amity."[14] He sees the shift to self-mutilation as a form of mental illness as at its core a moral panic, but in quite a different way: "It is as if the presence of a self-mutilator threatens the sense of mental or physical integrity of those around him or her."[15] For a practice that had been focused outward at the Other comes to be seen as an internal force aimed at the Self. For Favazza in 1987, there is a clear relationship between "culturally sanctioned and deviant self-mutilation"[16] They both are forms of the psychological "remediation" of "pathological conditions" ranging from epidemics to the "sexual rapaciousness of females" in a society.[17] They are forms of magical thinking. His examples of self-mutilation include the "saints who mortified their bodies in imitation of Jesus's suffering."[18] Yet he stresses that in 1987 the "most commonly encountered type of pathological self-mutilation is skin cutting by adolescents."[19] His readers might expect that the stigmata of the religiously fervent would be more frequently occurring, but Favazza aims to show that the real sufferers of this "pathology" are being overlooked. Favazza's view dominates the debates generated by in the moral panic about the "new epidemic" of adolescent cutting.

Such a view of self-harm was much in line with the tone that psychiatrists and historians took when they argued about anorexia nervosa up until the 1980s. It is only in the last thirty years or so that psychiatrists and historians alike have drawn a clear distinction between self-starvation by Central European saints in the middle ages and middle-class anorexia nervosa as a psychiatric category as defined by William Gull in 1873—namely that the two are *not* the same thing.[20] Yet Favazza, in a later publication, sees his undertaking in relation to anorexia: "Just as anorexia and bulimia nervosa did several years ago, self-mutilation is making its way into public consciousness."[21] His own work had the force of making this pattern popular, much as Hilde Bruch's writing made anorexia into a household word.

To offer a taste of this approach let us look at a follow-up essay by Favazza to his book. In a 1998 essay Favazza observes that

> certainly, self-mutilation has been around for a long time. In Book Six of the History, Herodotus (5th century B.C.) describes the actions of a deranged, probably psychotic, Spartan leader: 'As soon as the knife was in his hands, Cleomenes began to mutilate himself, beginning on his shins. He sliced his flesh into strips, working upward to his thighs, hips and sides until he reached his belly, which he chopped into mincemeat.[22]

Let us read Herodotus on Cleomenes in an older (non–"self-harm") translation:

> On his behaving thus, and showing that he was gone quite out of his mind, his kindred imprisoned him, and even put his feet in the stocks. While so bound, finding himself left alone with a single keeper, he asked the man for a knife. The keeper at first refused, whereupon Cleomenes began to threaten him, until at last he was afraid, being only a helot, and gave him what he required. Cleomenes had no sooner got the steel than, beginning at his legs, he horribly disfigured himself, cutting gashes in his flesh, along his legs, thighs, hips, and loins, until at last he reached his belly, which he likewise began to gash, whereupon in a little time he died.[23]

I am not using Favazza's translation here, as it clearly reflects his projection of self-harm into the world of universal "psychotic" behavior. But even Herodotus of Halicarnassus, who certainly does not like the Spartans, notes multiple possible causes for these "mad" acts in terms of ancient ideas of the possible etiologies of madness:

> The Greeks generally think that this fate came upon him because he induced the Pythoness to pronounce against Demaratus; the Athenians differ from all others in saying that it was because he cut down the sacred grove of the goddesses. The Argives say that Cleomenes lost his senses, and died so miserably, on account of these doings. But his own countrymen declare that his madness proceeded not from any supernatural cause whatever, but only from the habit of drinking wine unmixed with water, which he learnt of the Scyths.

Likewise, Favazza in his 1998 publication cites an 1846 essay by G. H. Bergmann as:

> the first published medical article on SM was a case report of a 48-year-old, manic-depressive widow who accused herself of being a great sinner. After walking naked in the street and asking various men, including her minister, to marry her, she was hospitalized. There she felt that her eyes were sinful. After reading Matthew's words in the Bible about plucking out an offensive eye, she enucleated both of hers and asked the doctor to cut off her legs and feet. She felt that because Christ shed his blood, she must shed hers to become saintly.[24]

Now terms such as "psychotic" and "manic depression" are those of twentieth-century clinical psychiatry and they "translate" the notions of the papers into language that may seem universal to the general reader of our day but which is indeed very period bound.

Victorian Self-Mutilation

If we look at some of the actual nineteenth century papers of self-mutilation, we can see quite a different rhetoric at work:

> It appears that the patient is a well-conducted servant girl, twenty-three years of age; she has light hair and complexion, and has been in service for the last nine months with a widow lady at Islington, where she never showed any signs of mental aberration. . . . On examination, it was found that the left hand had been severed from the arm as cleanly as a saw could have done it, the only difference with an ordinary amputation being, that no soft parts had been left for covering the lower ends of the radius and ulna, . . . It would appear that the bleeding was inconsiderable. . . . The patient seems to be strictly

> mono-maniac, as she gives very apposite and satisfactory answers respecting her age, state of health, family, and various other circumstances. When questioned, however, as to the unfortunate mutilation she has inflicted upon herself, she invariably answers that God told her to do it. When closely pressed as to how she knew that she ought to commit such an act, she appears wrapped in her monomania, and merely answers, "God knows."[25]

Neither manic depression nor psychosis is present. It is "monomania" as a partial insanity that is the illness that has self-mutilation as its symptom. And monomania in this form is very specifically a disease of adult women. Thus J. E. D. Esquirol amid the psychiatric revolution of his day defined monomania in 1838. This view of the monomanias included religious mania:

> Are not women under the control of influences to which men are strangers such as menstruation, pregnancy, confinement, and nursing? The passions, which among them are so active religion which is a veritable passion with many when love does not exclusively occupy their heart and mind jealousy fear do not these act more energetically upon the minds of than men. Religious melancholy is also very frequent among them in the lower classes of society and in countries where ignorance prevails. Girls, widows, and sometimes women at the critical period of life are a prey to erotic melancholy. Men, says Zimmermann, are insane from pride, girls from love, and women from jealousy.[26]

In his 1820 text *On Madness,* Etienne Georget earlier noted that "the religious fanatic is mild, he exhorts by casting his eyes at the heavens or fixing them on the earth. . . ."[27] But such a passive physiognomy is defined specifically as a quality of the feminine psyche even when found in men in contrast to the "the monomaniacal king [who] has a proud, inflated expression."

The clinical literature of the time seems to echo this view of religious monomania and self-harm, unless one is speaking of sexual self-mutilation. In an 1857 paper on "Extraordinary Self Mutilation" in *The Lancet,* this is seen as the quality of the masculine:

> . . . The man's shirt being almost through its whole extent besmeared with blood; this, however, proceeded from an extensive wound in the scrotum, the appearance of which, together with the answers I received to three or four questions of mine, led me to have the man removed to the hospital, when I lost no time in visiting him. On

> examining him more minutely than I had before, I found the left testicle protruding through the wound in the scrotum. . . . In early life he very frequently indulged in onanism, and to such an extent that when he attained the age of manhood he found himself almost impotent. In order to create sexual excitement, and subsequent masturbation, he tortured his imagination to devise means by which he might gratify his filthy passion. For a considerable time he was successful; but some five or six years ago he had again to tax his imaginative powers for some new method, and the idea struck him that the introduction of the point of a pen knife into the scrotum, and afterward some blunt instrument to titilate the testicles, (pour chatoullier les testicules,) might answer the purpose for a considerable period.[28]

The "monomanists" among the alienists define pain through self-harm as the gendered quality of the female. But it is a symptom that may help define a greater category of mental illness, not an illness in and of itself.

Now the debates about masculinity and pathology are not just to be found in Victorian medical literature. British society was roiled with the debate about the extension of civil rights to the Jews in the 1830s, which comes retrospectively to be seen as the great debate about circumcision as a sign of Jewish particularism. Can a circumcised Jew be an Englishman?[29] Genital self-mutilation as part of a vocabulary of cultural images is clear. It is a sign of the primitive as opposed to the civilized.

For Charles Darwin in *The Descent of Man* (1871), self-mutilation is universal but primitive. Its presentation, however, is not in the symbolic language of cutting and mutilating but in the propensity of "savages" to mutilation, claiming that "[h]ardly any part of the body, which can be unnaturally modified, has escaped."[30]

> As the face with us is chiefly admired for its beauty, so with savages it is the chief seat of mutilation. In all quarters of the world the septum, and more rarely the wings of the nose are pierced, with rings, sticks, feathers, and other ornaments inserted into the holes. The ears are everywhere pierced and similarly ornamented, and with the Botucudos and Lenguas of South America the hole is gradually so much enlarged that the lower edge touches the shoulder.[31]

Mutilation is self-harm in these examples, but there is no discourse of pain in this discussion, while Darwin is obsessed with pain elsewhere in his work.[32] Here self-harm is a question of male identity, and the pathological comes to be defined in terms of atavism. Drawing on the work of A. R. Wallace, Darwin also emphasized the value of the "social instincts" in the process of evolution by natural selection in man, while relating mutilation for the purposes of adornment directly to the "selfishness" that anthropologists such as E. B. Tylor saw as characteristic of "primitive" societies.[33]

> In most, but not all parts of the world, the men are more highly ornamented than the women, and often in a different manner; sometimes, though rarely, the women are hardly at all ornamented. As the women are made by savages to perform the greatest share of the work, and as they are not allowed to eat the best kinds of food, so it accords with the characteristic selfishness of man that they should not be allowed to obtain, or to use, the finest ornaments. Lastly it is a remarkable fact, as proved by the foregoing quotations, that the same fashions in modifying the shape of the head, in ornamenting the hair, in painting, tattooing, perforating the nose, lips, or ears, in removing or filing the teeth, &c., now prevail and have long prevailed in the most distant quarters of the world. It is extremely improbable that these practices which are followed by so many distinct nations are due to tradition from any common source. They rather indicate the close similarity of the mind of man, to whatever race he may belong, in the same manner as the almost universal habits of dancing, masquerading, and making rude pictures.[34]

Thus madness is a form of atavism. as Darwin had argued in *The Expression of Emotions in Men and Animals* (1872).[35] Self-mutilation is male and is a return to more primitive senses of the self.

Cesare Lombroso and Guglielmo Ferrero in their joint *The Female Offender* (1895) agree about self-mutilation, here in the form of tattooing, as a male and as an atavistic activity:

> Among male criminals the practice of tattooing is so common as to become a special characteristic but in female delinquents it is so rare as to be practically non-existent. Out of 1,175 sentenced women observed by me by Gamba and Salsotto only 13 or 215 per cent were tattooed. Among female lunatics the percentage is larger at any rate in Ancona where Riva found 10 tattooed out of 147 that is to say 68 per cent. All were tattooed on the arm and almost all the signs were either religious symbols such as seals or crosses or else they were dates. There were no images. One had on the arm a cross surmounting a globe with which she had been tattooed by a mountebank. Another had also on the arm self inflicted four initials being those of her mother and two lovers. This woman was a Venetian, an adulteress condemned for wounding her paramour

> and was affected with syphilis. Yet another Venetian woman had four initials on her arm.[36]

This view continues in criminology well into the 1950s, where tattooing and criminality remain intimately related.[37] Now it is clear that even Darwin and Lombroso did not necessarily see tattooing as self-mutilation in the same sense that Victorian clinicians saw castration or enucleating. Yet it is a symptom or sign for an anthropological reading of self-mutilation. It indicates a throwback to an earlier state of development. There seems to be no specific references in the Victorian clinical literature, for example, to tattooing as a symptom of self-harm. Yet the border between the idea of an atavistic model for madness and the use of the symptom of self-mutilation as an index for madness is certainly present.

In the Victorian medical world, in the moral panic about self-harm these worlds collide. Thus "all the states of mind leading to self-mutilation, self-torture, &c., hitherto considered, are compatible with reputed sanity, although they are to insanity near akin, and generally indicate more or less mental derangement."[38] Such self-mutilation deals with notions of sexual self-harm, therefore are concerns for a society that is focused on ideas of a healthy masculinity. In 1897, the popular view is that "self-mutilation in man is almost invariably the result of meditation over the generative function, and the great majority of cases of this nature are avulsions or amputations of some parts of the genitalia."[39] As Sarah Chaney has recently shown by

> examining the prevalence of the behaviours considered "self-mutilation" at the Bethlem Royal Hospital between 1880 and 1900, castration hardly registers—just three male patients (out of a total of around two thousand) within this period attempted self-castration, and one further threatened it. In contrast, seventeen patients attempted to pluck out their eyes, while every year more than four patients picked their faces, pulled out their hair or knocked their heads against the wall (Bethlem Royal Hospital Patient Casebooks, 1880–1900).[40]

In other words, the world of the nineteenth century focuses on specific forms of self-mutilation and fits them into preformed ideas of mental illness. Such cases are merely the Victorian medical parallel to the Victorian obsession with the self-mutilation of the primitive and as such are proof of the very atavistic nature of insanity. They are not "typical," as Chaney argues, but exemplary of the radical nature of the mad as throwbacks. Yet still they remain only symptoms and are never given the status of being seen as a disease process in and of itself.

Cutting and Sexuality in the Age of Psychoanalysis

The earliest sexologists such as Heinrich Kaan in 1844 observed that self-harm and the self-indulgence in pain is the quality of a specific subgroup:

> In individuals suffering oversensitivity there are various pains: pain of rheumatism, face pain come into sight, in the production and maintenance of these this psychopathology contributed not a little: all of these diseases are more unique to the wealthy, in whom certainly the aberration of the sexual instinct occurs more frequently than amongst the poor. Familiar pains come into evidence at home, less in the hospital, always in association with an apathy of the entire sexual life.[41]

The luxury of pain, for Kaan, is the result of class, not gender. Yet early on, pain and male sexuality becomes a symptom of the definition of sexual obsession as "masochism." Richard Krafft-Ebing's *Psychopathia sexualis* (1886) creates "masochism" as the perverse desire to experience control (not necessarily inflict pain) by the sexual object. He says, "the extreme consequences of masochism, however, are checked by the instinct of self-preservation, and therefore murder and serious injury, which may be committed in sadistic excitement, have here in reality, so far as known, no passive equivalent."[42] The "passive" mode would be the feminine as it is not an accident that Krafft-Ebing's model for the masochist, as is noted even in his own time, is *Venus in Furs*, a novella by Austrian author Leopold von Sacher-Masoch, published in 1870. Male masochism is postulated as contrary to the inherently aggressive nature of male sexuality. Thus pain aimed at the self—whether self-induced as in self-harm or induced by a partner (as in sadomasochism) is a paraphilia.

The idea of harm and self-harm is present in an attenuated manner in Sigmund Freud's *Three Essays on Sexuality* (1905): "it has also been claimed that every pain contains in itself the possibility of a pleasurable sensation. Let us be satisfied with the impression that the explanation of this perversion is by no means satisfactory and that it is possible that many psychic efforts unite themselves into one effect."[43] Masochism "comprises any passive attitude towards sexual life and the sexual object, the extreme instance of which appears to be that in which satisfaction is conditional upon suffering physical or mental pain at the hands of the sexual object."[44] He continues, "Pain, which is overridden in such cases, thus falls into line with disgust and shame as a force that stands in opposition and resistance to the libido. Sadism and masochism occupy a special position among the perversions, since the contrast between activity and passivity which lies behind them is among the universal characteristics of sexual life."[45] It is universal and may have an evolutionary source, but one very different from Darwin's notion of self-mutilation. It may be "a relic of cannibalistic desires—that is, it is a contribution derived from the apparatus for obtaining mastery, which is concerned with the satisfaction of the other and, ontogenetically, the older of the great instinctual needs. It has also been maintained that every pain contains in itself the possibility of a feeling of pleasure."[46] For Freud there is a distinction between primary and secondary masochism. Primary masochism relates to the death drive (*Todestrieb*) and manifests itself in true self-abasement in regard to rejection by the desired object. Secondary masochism is "merely" the enacted role of rejection and punishment by the masochist who knows that this is the result of a mutually agreed upon contract that defines the roles as roles. For Freud the latter may be a form of acceptable playacting (and so Gilles Deleuze reads Severin in Sacher-Masoch's tale), while the former is a debasement of the male sexual role.

Masochism is not monomania, as monomania is feminine and masochism is inherently masculine. Neither category evokes "class" as does Kaan, yet the case material for monomania is almost exclusively working class, as is that for male sexual mutilation. Severin in Sacher Masoch's tale may be the exception, but his class identity is vague. The idea of a distinction between the male and the female experience of and articulation of self-harm is thus part of nineteenth-century pathologization of self-harm within clinical psychiatry and beyond. But Freud's idea of self-harm has its roots as well in the evolutionary theory of the day.

By the twentieth century, self-harm has begun to shift meaning. Under the impact of psychoanalytic theory (and Freud's views of masochism), the model of what constitutes self-harm shifts. Cutting rather than sexual self-abasement or self-mutilation becomes the symptom that will define this new reading of self-mutilation. In a paper from 1913 we are introduced to "the patient [who] was a young woman twenty-three years old. She came to the Hospital with a self-inflicted cut on her left arm. Her arm had many other scars, and there was one on her breast: she said she had cut herself twenty-eight or thirty times; and on the calf of her right leg was a scar forming the letter W."[47] The psychoanalyst is confronted with "Two problems [that] presented themselves: Why did she cut herself? How could she be helped?" We have moved from the world of the Victorian clinical image of self-mutilation to the world of psychoanalytic cutting.

Yet in the background the boundary between cutting and other forms of body modification remains tenuous. Darwin's view of self-mutilation as a pathological sign of atavism remains associated even with socially more acceptable forms. In 1925 an analyst observes "the crazy exhibitionism of tattooing may have one of its origins in the exercise of the driving urge to self-torture, what I have called the suicidal-tendency; to create the awe of superiority by proving one's capacity for excessive pain. The element of display, is contributory and derivative, it seems to me."[48] This picks up a thread in Freud's work on the analogy between primitive and neurotic mentality of 1913, in which he notes the potential origin of totemism in tattooing.[49] Here too it is always necessary, as Karl A. Menninger observes in a paper on "Localized Self-Destruction: Self-Mutilations" as a form of self destruction in 1934 notes to explain "customary and conventional forms of such as ear piercing, trimming the nails, hair cutting and shaving . . . from the standpoint of unconscious motivation"[50] They are a form of attenuated and socially acceptable self-mutilation; cutting is neither attenuated nor socially acceptable.

Psychoanalytic practice focuses on self-harm as symptom—but not of an atavistic madness but as a problem in self-awareness and self-construction. As Elizabeth Lunbeck notes, this seemed to be "registered the demise of the Freudian patient with her classic neuroses and specific symptoms and the ascendancy of the chronically maladapted, character disordered new patient."[51] Thus Thomas Szasz says in 1957 not about tattooing or "cutting" but about radical self-mutilation, "the actual removal of parts of the body by the patient":

> The lack of affect vis-a-vis the body corresponds to, and is the converse of, the hypochondriacal preoccupations with the body. The former expresses the affect appropriate to the fait accompli of body loss, just as the latter corresponds to a hypercathexis of the body. The foregoing state occasionally leads to the actual removal of parts of the body by the patient. This expresses the ego's need to bring the body up to date, so to speak, in order that it should correspond to the psychically amputated (new) body image. Since the body part was already lost from the point of view of the experiencing ego, its removal is *unaccompanied by pain.* On the contrary, successful self-mutilation leads to a feeling of work well done: ". . . in all cases the event was accompanied by a feeling of relief and tranquility and there were no regrets." (Hemphill) This is understandable if we compare the feeling or experience of no longer existing (e.g., the body is dead) described above, to an unwanted memory [such as that of a loved (needed) and

> mourned person]. Implicit in such a memory is the remembrance of a previous state different from the one at present and a (conscious) confrontation of these two experiences.[52]

The description is similar to but not identical to that of the nineteenth-century clinical self-mutilator, but the emphasis is on the psychic qualities of relief rather than on the radical physical mutilation and its implications. The emphasis is on the decoupling of the mutilation and pain as part of a psychic chain of dissociation. Louis A. Sass situated this in the world of the 1960s and '70s, where:

> Only through imagining this kind of lived-world can one begin to understand how schizophrenics could be capable of performing certain real-world actions that, to the normal person, would be unimaginably horrible. In extreme cases, such patients may seriously mutilate themselves—even, for example, cutting off their own genitals or putting out their eyes. Though their sensory organs still function and they are cognitively aware of their actions, they do not appear to experience any pain or to register the significance and irreversibility of what they have done. When one talks to these patients, it almost seems that, for them, everything involved in the action—the body part, the cutting, even the pain itself—is a purely theoretical phenomenon, as if the action had been but a thought experiment, a removal of idea-of-penis or idea-of-eye rather than the actual organ of flesh, blood, and screaming nerve. Many schizophrenic patients often do feel separated from the lived-body: "Body and soul don't belong together; there's no unity," stated one of Manfred Bleuler's patients.[53]

Mutilation is a form of abstraction of the body, reducing it to its theoretical implications rather than being seen as divine or sexual. But over and over again, the clinical focus is on severe self-mutilation, not cutting.

Thus cutting is placed in an equivalent but lesser position to severe self-mutilation. In the mid-twentieth century, self-harm seems to be found in a world constituted by various images of mutilation, but cutting is always present, as in the popular psychoanalytic account by Marguerite Sechehaye in the 1950s:

> The orders, or rather impulses, persuaded me to harm myself. I bit my hands, my arms, cruelly; I beat my head against the wall; I struck my chest so hard with my fist I was covered with bruises and it was necessary to protect *me* from myself. An inconceivable urge to destruction rose in me, an urge to annihilate myself at all costs. And I was profoundly guilty, a guilt vast and horrible, unbearable,

> remorseless; of what I knew not, yet deeply, immeasurably guilty. I would not eat; by any means I tried to destroy myself. Only Mama was able to prevent it.[54]

In the course of the next thirty years the importance of the symptom of cutting is enhanced and eventually becomes the focus of clinical attention.

Borderline

The psychoanalytic contexts are important because by the 1950s self-harm was beginning to become a symptom, not of masochism or psychosis, but of borderline personality disorder, the hot, new psychiatric category inspired by postwar psychiatry and its integration of psychoanalytic views of self-harm.

In 1968, the *Diagnostic and Statistical Manual of the American Psychiatric Association-II* attempted to standardize psychiatric classification in line with the International Classification of Diseases (ICD). In 1974, Robert L. Spitzer was assigned to revise DSM-II and bring it in line with the newest medical (read: somatic) theories of mental illness. Spitzer examined the unreliable classifications of DSM-II and demanded new and specific diagnostic criteria for the medical diagnosis of mental illness. DSM-III thus came into being. This was the first truly systematic rethinking of mental illness in the age in which the emerging field of the genetics of mental illness and the broader introduction of psychotropic drugs in the treatment of mental illness came to define psychiatric theory and practice. The psychoanalytic assumptions of DSM-II seemed to have been generally abandoned, and a new science of psychiatry appeared. Despite this apparent abandonment, psychoanalytic assumptions underpinned much of DSM-III.

We can see the end product of this integration in 1980, when borderline personality disorder first appears in the *Diagnostic and Statistical Manual of the American Psychiatric Association-III*. The vagueness of the category is acknowledged, but "frequently there is impulsive and unpredictable behavior that is potentially physically self-damaging." The acts are defined as "suicidal gestures, self-mutilation, recurrent accidents or physical fights."[55] It is "apparently common" but "more commonly diagnosed in women."[56] In *Diagnostic and Statistical Manual of the American Psychiatric Association-IV* (1994), self-injuring behavior is present as criterion 5 of borderline personality disorder (301.83): "Recurrent suicidal behavior, gestures, or thoughts or self-mutilating behavior." Borderline comes to define the new idea of self-mutilating behavior as a metaphor made physically concrete. The World Health Organization's

International Statistical Classification of Diseases and Related Health Problems, 10th Revision (known as "ICD-10") (1993) defines "F60.31 Borderline type" as manifesting itself in "acts of self-harm."

Elizabeth Lunbeck argues that while borderline personality disorder phenomena were documented by clinical psychiatrists, Borderline Personality Disorder was the result of "the fitful coalescence of a new category—assembled from new concepts and new terms—that has enabled clinicians to take note of and diagnose dimensions of personhood they had not formerly been able or inclined to register."[57] Borderline personality disorder evolved in the United States over the twentieth century as a category that identified patients who "fit frankly neither in the psychotic nor into the psychoneurotic group," and conventional wisdom was that "this border-line group of patients is extremely difficult to handle."[58] This image of the new "borderline" patient is from a paper by Adolf Stern in 1938. Following Stern's observation, Helene Deutsch described a lack of subjective experience of distress in a group of patients with "as-if" personalities.[59] In 1953, psychoanalyst Robert Knight acknowledged the "wastebasket," poorly defined, catchall nature, of the borderline diagnosis, that reappears in the DSM-III definition. In Knight's view, the diagnosis meant that "a patient is quite sick but not frankly psychotic" in nomenclature and reflected clinicians' anxiety facing treatment with a patient who presented severe symptoms that were otherwise hard to characterize, let alone treat.[60]

By the 1970s, "borderline" had become a diagnostic category in clinical psychiatry as well, and self-harm became one of the defining symptoms. Otto Kernberg stressed that self-harm is to be found within the borderline personality organization, which is a "specific, stable, pathological personality organization." Kernberg defines borderline from the perspective of ego psychology with its concern for separation-individuation but also with a deep acknowledgment of its instinctual underpinnings. Kernberg also defines what he calls the "presumptive symptoms" of borderline, from diffuse anxiety, "polysymptomatic neurosis"— multiple phobias, to impulsivity and addiction. He also mentions what he (in an odd way following Darwin) calls "Primitive Self-destructiveness."

> There exists a "low level" group of masochistic characters, in which rather primitive sexualization of masochistic needs occurs, masochistic perverse trends may be present, and aggression is discharged indiscriminately toward the outside or toward one's own body. Patients with severe self-destructiveness (but without a well-integrated

> superego and with a remarkable absence of the capacity to experience guilt) are members of this group. Typical examples are provided by patients who obtain nonspecific relief of anxiety by cutting themselves or by some other form of self-mutilation, or by impulsive suicidal gestures carried out with great rage and practically no depression.[61]

Later he undertakes a much more detailed account of the subtypes of self-mutilation among Borderline patients that:

> illustrate a most primitive type of self-destructiveness with conscious or unconscious pleasure connected with the pain they inflict on themselves, a severity of aggression directed against themselves that is neither centered in superego pathology (an unconscious sense of guilt) nor directly linked with erotic strivings (or at least, such erotic strivings occupy a very secondary role to that of aggressive impulses).[62]

These symptoms of self-mutilation are never the defining moment for the classification of the borderline patient.

Yet self-harm comes to be seen more and more as an autonomous diagnostic category as it is defined beyond the boundary of borderline personality disorder. In 1983 Joel Kahan and E. Mansell Pattison coined the term "deliberate self-harm syndrome," which included the irresistible impulse to self-harm, a sense of psychological entrapment, increasing affective response to such entrapment, cognitive constriction of alternatives, repetitive private, self destructive acts, and a resultant sense of relief as characteristic symptoms.[63] Their claim was that the

> analysis of 56 published case reports of self-harm revealed a typical pattern of onset in late adolescence, multiple recurrent episodes, low lethality, harm deliberately inflicted upon the body, and extension of the behavior over many years. The 4 predominant psychological symptoms for this syndrome are despair, anxiety, anger, and cognitive constriction. Predisposing factors include lack of social support, homosexuality (in men), drug and alcohol abuse, and suicidal ideation (in women).[64]

They strongly proposed a category for DSM-IV, which was not accepted, claiming "the deliberate self-harm syndrome is a specific clinical subset different from the clinical subset of suicidal behavior."[65] Self-harm in their definition seems to be focused in the sixteen-to-twenty-five-year-old group and was clearly not gender neutral, as it was seen as more often present in women and gay men. The refusal to consider this as a DSM-IV category left self-harm in the 1980s as a symptom recognized as existing within a specific diagnostic category (borderline) but not yet as an autonomous diagnosis.

The New Self-Harm

In the early twenty-first century, self-harm transcends its use in the earlier discussions of borderline. Kernberg's borderline patients tended to be seen as both socially self-destructive as well as physically self-harming. But self-harm is for him a peripheral symptom. With the rise of trauma theory in the 1990s, such cases are now more and more defined in terms of self-harm as an independent diagnostic category.[66] And the etiology of self-harm reflects early childhood trauma:

> The cause of self-harm overwhelmingly points to childhood trauma, with sexual abuse and lack of secure attachments the leading culprits. The trauma history of a patient who engages in self-harm is as accurately pathognomonic as a radiograph is of a Pouteau fracture.[67]

Self-harm is in this view a primary diagnostic category rather than a peripheral symptom. Indeed, it comes to be seen as an autonomous category.

The new feminism clearly foregrounds self-harm as an autonomous category. Thus Elizabeth Grosz sees cutting as aggression turned inward. She defines the body as an "inscriptive surface" reflecting both intrapsychic and cultural forces. Grosz describes more self-harm as part of a "social inscription that bind all subjects."[68] Self-harm reflects how "culturally specific grids of power, regulation, and force" distort the psyche.[69] But the scars also label her as noncompliant.[70] Thus there is an attempt to rehabilitate the self-cutter (much as 1970s feminism attempted to rehabilitate the hysteric as speaking in the true voice of the feminine in the works of Monique Wittig, Helene Cixous, and Gayatri Spivak):

> A profusion of officially recognised names for self-harm including: "deliberate self-injury," "self-inflicted violence," "self attack," "self-cutting," "deliberate nonfatal act," and "symbolic wounding." But many of these names are subject to dispute on the grounds that they fail to hear the voice of the self-cut skin . . . or that they represent a hostile response to it.[71]

Self-cutting is a reasonable response to an irrational world.

These views parallel the alternative views of insanity in the 1960s in the works of Erving Goffman, R. D. Laing, and Thomas Szasz (the latter of which had a powerful impact on feminism and gay rights), where inherently different theories of the etiology and meaning of insanity come to be seen as examining the social causes of mental illness. Feminist debates view cutting as a positive act or as a marker of the repressive patriarchy. Where in the 1960s Goffman saw the asylum as a repressive means of social control, Szasz saw madness as invented by the patient as well as society and Laing saw it as the "healthy" product of sick social or familial structures. Critical disability and feminist embodiment theories redefine the meanings of borderline stigmata, such as scars from cutting, and redefine cutting as an embodied and material discursive practice. The irony is that such an approach reincorporates socially acceptable forms of body modification, such as tattooing, into the broader category now labeled as "body-marking." Kay Inckle coins this term:

> to incorporate the bodily interventions that are normally described as either "self-injury" or body modification. I use a single term in order to firstly, explore the links between embodied practices which are expressed through body alteration and, secondly, to critique the binaries of definition that are reiterated within normative terminology.[72]

All are the same, and all are to be read as positive in their expressiveness. It simply reverses the model now incorporating all forms of body-marking as means of healthy self-expression.

The moral panic about cutting as a psychopathological category is also present in its reversal and now defines the very nature of self-harm. Its cultural significance is such that while both psychoanalytically informed and clinical psychiatry in the post–WWII world were concerned with such self-destructive activities, it was never seen as a major factor in mental health. By 2011 the question of self-harm has reached the mainstream of American psychiatry. And it is so present in popular culture as to generate a positive rereading of it as a standalone diagnostic category. In the newest version of DSM-5, published in May 2013, self-harm is now become its own diagnostic category, nonsuicidal self-injury:

> A. In the last year, the individual has, on 5 or more days, engaged in intentional self-inflicted damage to the surface of his or her body of a sort likely to induce bleeding, bruising, or pain (e.g., cutting, burning, stabbing, hitting, excessive rubbing), with the expectation that the injury will lead to only minor or moderate physical harm (i.e., there is no suicidal intent). **Note:** The absence of suicidal intent has either been stated by the individual or can be inferred by the individual's repeated engagement in a behavior that the individual knows, or has learned, is not likely to result in death.

B. The individual engages in the self-injurious behavior with one or more of the following expectations:
   1. To obtain relief from a negative feeling or cognitive state.
   2. To resolve an interpersonal difficulty.
   3. To induce a positive feeling state.
   Note: The desired relief or response is experienced during or shortly after the self-injury, and the individual may display patterns of behavior suggesting a dependence on repeatedly engaging in it.

C. The intentional self-injury is associated with at least one of the following:
   1. Interpersonal difficulties or negative feelings or thoughts, such as depression, anxiety, tension, anger, generalized distress, or self-criticism, occurring in the period immediately prior to the self-injurious act.
   2. Prior to engaging in the act, a period of preoccupation with the intended behavior that is difficult to control.
   3. Thinking about self-injury that occurs frequently, even when it is not acted upon.

D. The behavior is not socially sanctioned (e.g., body piercing, tattooing, part of a religious or cultural ritual) and is not restricted to picking a scab or nail biting.

E. The behavior or its consequences cause clinically significant distress or interference in interpersonal, academic, or other important areas or functioning.

F. The behavior does not occur exclusively during psychotic episodes, delirium, substance intoxication, or substance withdrawal. In individuals with a neurodevelopmental disorder, the behavior is not part of a pattern of repetitive stereotypies. The behavior is not better explained by another mental disorder or medical condition (e.g., psychotic disorder, autism spectrum disorder, intellectual disability, Lesch-Nyhan syndrome, stereotypic movement disorder with self-injury, trichotillomania [hair-pulling disorder], excoriation [skin-picking] disorder).

   The behavior does not occur exclusively during states of psychosis, delirium, or intoxication. In individuals with a developmental disorder, the behavior is not part of a pattern of repetitive stereotopies. The behavior cannot be accounted for by another mental or medical disorder (i.e., psychotic disorder, pervasive developmental disorder, mental retardation, Lesch-Nyhan Syndrome).[73]

These behaviors are now to be understood as the basis for a diagnosis of treatable mental disorder.

New Boundaries?

With the publication of DSM-5, the moral panic about cutting has moved self-harm (in this limited sense) to the fore as a standalone diagnostic category, something quite impossible in the 1980s. The newest idea of self-harm now clearly brackets those actions that are not socially sanctioned: self-mutilation is a symptom but not a sanctioned social practice. Yet in 2012, it is not just tattooing and piercing that are socially sanctioned; the contemporary definition of acceptable bodily transformation now includes a wide range of surgical alteration, piercing, and augmentation of the genitalia as well as the tattooing of the cornea and piercing of the eyeball (extraocular implants). We can bracket: Darwin and Lombroso on tattooing as well as much of the Victorian literature on male sexual self-mutilation and female self-mutilation.

Self-mutilation is also not the product of any self-destructive action of psychosis of any form. Thus all of the concerns about monomania and self-mutilation vanish from our twenty-first-century milieu. Self-injury must be associated with a mental state such as "depression, anxiety, tension, anger, generalized distress, or self-criticism," but this scale seems to run from a diagnostic category in DSM-5 (depression) to one that at best may well be a form of a healthy mental state (self-criticism). And self-harm must be at the same time repetitive (a preoccupation) if only in desire rather than in action. This variant on the idea of suicidal ideation makes the very idea of self-cutting into a marker. One of the strongest movements in nineteenth-century psychiatry (and with Emil Durkheim, nineteenth-century sociology) was to brand all suicide as psychopathological.[74] We can thus eliminate: nineteenth-century views of self-mutilation as the result of mental illnesses of all etiologies, as one does not actually have to have done the act prior to being potentially diagnosed as self-harming. It is enough to have thought about it obsessively.

Self-harm is limited in its form to those actions that cause blood to flow either subcutaneously or visibly and are painful. But it does not extend to self-amputation or any attempt to violate the body that could potentially be construed as suicidal (i.e., the shallow cutting of the wrists with limited blood loss) even if this action does not lead to imminent danger of loss of life. Here again, new definitions require setting aside all of the psychoanalytic theories that decoupled self-harm and pain and stressed psychic origins in earlier states of development or psychic experience. The new self-mutilation is quotidian. It is measured by daily events and daily repetition. It is neither part of the social fabric nor is it a symptom of forms of acute mental illness. It is thus not a sign of suicidal intent even though it is defined as a mental state prior to any self-harming action.

The question that DSM-5 asks us is not whether we are much further today then we were with earlier boundary setting concerning acceptable and unacceptable, socially bounded and symptomatic self-harm. But rather, how is it that the most recent moral panic about self-harm set its boundaries? (I do not exclude the fact that most of the concern in the nineteenth century with self-harm was already a form of moral panic.) Self-harm is not socially sanctioned; it is a taboo act. What happens when it is socially sanctioned in the form of body piercing and tattooing? Does the associated pain become a secondary effect? If the goals attendant to today's self-mutilation are to cause specific somatic manifestations, such as bleeding or bruising or pain, how do we separate out these experiences? For all are attendant to those forms of (Darwinian) self-mutilation that are socially sanctioned. If the focus is on the fact that self-mutilation impacts on the course of daily life and excludes other mental or social activities, is it then as a form of obsessive-compulsive disorder? Just as one person's religion is another's religious mania in the age of Victoria, so is obsessiveness—is the limit well past those individuals who have body piercing, tattoos, and transdermal inserts to remake themselves in the visible form of reptiles (such as Erik Sprague, "The Lizardman," with sharpened teeth, full-body tattoo of green scales, bifurcated tongue, and recently, green-inked lips) or cats (such as Dennis Avner, "Cat Man," with tattooing, piercing of his upper lip and transdermal implants on his forehead to facilitate the wearing of whiskers, and flattening of his nose via septum relocation, among a range of other changes). The philosopher Ian Hacking, in an essay on the appearance of DSM-5, writes: "And trying to get it right, in revision after revision, [DSM] perpetuates the long-standing idea that, in our present state of knowledge, the recognized varieties of mental illness should neatly sort themselves into tidy blocks, in the way that plants and animals do."[75] But it is even more insidious than this. For by turning symptoms into diseases, the DSM reifies both the symptom and the disease, rather than grounding them in the moment when each becomes the concern of a society focusing on mental illness and mental health.

Remember my paradox at the very beginning of this piece: "A patient comes to you with the following complaint. 'I am very unhappy with my left leg. I have always been unhappy with it. It causes me constant unhappiness. I wish to have it removed.'" What do you do with actions that could result in death but result only in self-harm? If, according to the Israeli psychoanalyst Carlos Strenger, "Generation X" is the generation of the "designer self," then tattoos and body piercing come to be a sign of the desire and the ability of that generation to remake their body as a means of releasing tension and giving pleasure. Not a pathology at all, but a sign of the time and its attendant refashioning of the border between the "pathological" and the "normal."[76] The line today runs between "cutting" and "piercing."

Notes

1. See my *Making the Body Beautiful: A Cultural History of Aesthetic Surgery* (Princeton: Princeton University Press, 1999).
2. See Josephine Johnston and Carl Elliott, "Healthy limb amputation: ethical and legal aspects," *Clinical Medicine, Journal of the Royal College of Physicians*, 2 (2002): 431–435.
3. Ilana Löwy, *Preventative Strikes: Women, Precancer, and Prophylactic Surgery* (Baltimore; The Johns Hopkins University Press, 2010).
4. David W. Freeman "Self-harm shown common in teens: Why do they do it?" CBS News, November 21, 2011, cbsnews.com/news/self-harm-shown-common-in-teens-why-do-they-do-it/ (accessed November 18, 2013).
5. Stacey Chia, "Teen cutters now more discreet; Troubled youth cut themselves in less-visible areas, making it harder to get help to them," *The Straits Times Singapore*, November 6, 2011, p. 1.
6. Anonymous, "Center provides resources, help for self-mutilation." *India Pharma News*, July 22, 2011, p. 2.
7. Anonymous, "THE SPIRIT OF STOKES: Bringing them out of bondage: Exodus Ministries prepares for Open House on Saturday," *The Stokes News*, Walnut Cove, NC (June 23, 2011).
8. For example, Cheryl A. Rainfield, *Scars* (Lodi, NJ: WestSide Books, 2010), described by the publisher as the story of "Fifteen-year-old Kendra, a budding artist, has not felt safe since she began to recall devastating memories of childhood sexual abuse, especially since she cannot remember her abuser's identity, and she copes with the pressure by cutting herself." Or Julia Hoban, *Willow* (New York: Listening Library, 2009): "Sixteen-year-old Willow, who was driving the car that killed both of her parents, copes with the pain and guilt by cutting herself, until she meets a smart and sensitive boy who is determined to help her stop." Or the graphic novel: Tracy A. White, *How I Made it to Eighteen: A Mostly True Story* (New York: Roaring Brook Press, 2010.): "How do you know if you're on the verge of a nervous breakdown? For seventeen-year-old Stacy Black, it all begins with the smashing of a window. After putting her fist through the glass, she checks into a mental hospital. Stacy hates it there but despite herself slowly realizes she has to

face the reasons for her depression to stop from self-destructing. Based on the author's experiences, *How I Made it to Eighteen* is a frank portrait of what it's like to struggle with self-esteem, body image issues, drug addiction, and anxiety."

9. Armando R. Favazza, "The Coming of Age of Self-mutilation," *Journal of Nervous and Mental Diseases* 186 (1998): 259–68.
10. Armando R. Favazza, *Bodies under Siege: Self-mutilation and Body Modification in Culture and Psychiatry* (Baltimore: Johns Hopkins University Press, 1987).
11. Stanley Cohen, *Folk Devils and Moral Panics* (London: Macgibbon and Kee, 1972), here 9. Cohen did not coin this phrase. It first appeared in Jock Young, "The Role of the Police as Amplifiers of Deviance, Negotiators of Drug Control as Seen in Notting Hill," in Stanley Cohen, ed., *Images of Deviance* (Harmondsworth, England: Penguin, 1971), 27–61, and has since been used to analyze social "epidemics" such as "child abuse" and the "war on drugs."
12. Rachel Cottam, "Obesity and Culture," *The Lancet* 364, no. 9441 (2004): 1201–1203.
13. Favazza, *Bodies under Siege*, 1–60.
14. Ibid., 191.
15. Ibid., xii.
16. Ibid., 191.
17. Ibid., 191.
18. Ibid., 192.
19. Ibid., 193.
20. Or at least since Joan Brumberg, *Fasting Girls: The History of Anorexia Nervosa* (Cambridge: Harvard University Press, 1988). See also Richard A. Gordon, *Eating Disorders: Anatomy of a Social Epidemic* (Oxford: Blackwell Publishers, 2000); Marcia K. Ove, "The Evolution of Self-Starvation Behaviors into the Present-Day Diagnosis of Anorexia Nervosa: A Critical Literature Review," (PhD diss., California School of Professional Psychology, 2002) and Sherman Apt Russell, *Hunger: An Unnatural History* (New York: Basic Books, 2005).
21. Favazza, "Coming of Age."
22. Favazza, "Coming of Age."
23. *Herodotus*, Vol. II, ed., Arthur James Grant, trans., George Rawlinson (New York: C. Scribner's, 1897), 35. See also G. E. R. Lloyd, *In the grip of disease: studies in the Greek imagination* (Oxford: Oxford University Press, 2003), 133.
24. Favazza, "Coming of Age," quoting G. H. Bergmann "Ein Fall von religiöser Monomanie," *Algemeine Zeitschrift für Psychiatrie* 3 (1846): 365–380.
25. Lloyd, "St. Bartholomew's Hospital: Religious Monomania; Self-mutilation," *The Lancet* 58, no. 1472 (1851): 456.
26. Jean Étienne Dominique Esquirol, *Mental Maladies*, trans. E. K. Hunt (1838; repr. Philadelphia: Blanchard & Lea, 1845), 211.
27. Jean Etienne Georget, *De la folie* (Paris: Crevot, 1820), 133.
28. Anonymous, "Jersey Hospital: Extraordinary Self Mutilation," *The Lancet* 70, no. 1769 (1857): 88–89.
29. Todd Endelman, *The Jews of Georgian England, 1714–1830: Tradition and Change in a Liberal Society* (Ann Arbor: The University of Michigan Press, 1999).

30. Charles Darwin, *The Descent of Man, and Selection in Relation to Sex,* (London: John Murray, 1871), 342.
31. Darwin, 341.
32. See my "Seeing Bodies in Pain: From Hippocrates to Freud," *International Journal of Psychoanalysis* 92, no. 3: 661–674.
33. E. B. Tylor, "Primitive Society (Part I)," *Contemporary Review* 21 (1872): 701–718.
34. Darwin, 343.
35. Charles Darwin, *The Expression of Emotions in Men and Animals* (London: John Murray, 1872).
36. Cesare Lombroso and Guglielmo Ferrero, *The Female Offender* (London: Fisher Unwin, 1895), 115.
37. Hans von Hentig, *The Criminal and his Victim. Studies in the Sociobiology of Crime* (New Haven: Yale University Press, 1948).
38. James Adam, "Self-Mutilation," in *A Dictionary of Psychological Medicine,* ed., Daniel Hack Tuke (London: J. & A. Churchill, 1892) 1147–1152, here 1148.
39. George M. Gould, and Walter L. Pyle, *Anomalies and Curiosities of Medicine* (London: Rebman Publishing Co., 1897), 732.
40. Sarah Chaney, "'A Hideous Torture on Himself': Madness and Self-Mutilation in Victorian Literature," *Journal of Medical Humanities* 32 (2011): 279–289.
41. Quoted from the unpublished translation of Heinrich Kaan's *Psychopathia Sexualis* (Leipzig: Leopold Voss, 1844) by Benjamin Kahan.
42. Richard Krafft-Ebing, *Psychopathia Sexualis: With Especial Reference To Contrary Sexual Instinct,* trans., Charles Gilbert Chaddock (Philadelphia: F.A. Davis, 1892), 116.
43. Sigmund Freud, *Three Essays on the Theory of Sexuality, In Standard Edition of the Complete Psychological Works of Sigmund Freud,* ed. and trans. James Strachey, Anna Freud, Alix Strachey, and Alan Tyson. 24 vols. London: Hogarth, 1955–74, cited as SE, here Vol. VII (1905), 157.
44. Freud, SE, *Three Essays,* 157.
45. Ibid., 158.
46. Ibid., 158.
47. L. E. Emerson, "The Case of Miss A: A Preliminary Report of a Psychoanalytic Study and Treatment of a Case of Self-Mutilation," *Psychoanalytic Review* 1 (1913): 41–54.
48. Samuel D. Schmalhausen, "Psychoanalytic Studies," *Psychoanalytic Review* 12 (1925): 295–315, here 295.
49. Sigmund Freud, *Totem and Taboo: Some Points of Agreement between the Mental Lives of Savages and Neurotics* (1913 [1912–13]), *SE,* Vol. XIII (1913–1914), 108.
50. Karl A. Menninger, "Localized Self-Destruction: Self-Mutilations," *Psychoanalytic Quarterly* 3 (1934): 495–498, here, 496.
51. Elizabeth Lunbeck, "Borderline Histories: Psychoanalysis Inside and Out," *Science in Context* 19 (2006): 151–173.
52. Thomas Szasz, "The Psychology of Bodily Feelings in Schizophrenia," *Psychosomatic Medicine* 19 (1957): 11–16.

53. Louis A. Sass, *Paradoxes of Delusion: Wittgenstein, Schreber, and the Schizophrenic Mind* (Ithaca: Cornell university Press, 1994), 48, where he is referencing Manfred Bleuler, *The Schizophrenic Disorders* (1978), 490.
54. Marguerite Sechehaye, *Autobiography of a Schizophrenic Girl: The True Story of "Renee,"* trans. Grace Rubin-Rabson (New York City: Grune & Stratton, 1950).
55. *Diagnostic and Statistical Manual of Mental Disorders* (Third Edition) (Washington: American Psychiatric Association, 1980), 321–23.
56. DSM-III, 322.
57. Lunbeck, "Borderline Histories," 153.
58. Adolf Stern, "Psychoanalytic Investigation of and Therapy in the Border Line Group of Neuroses," *Psychoanalytic Quarterly*, 7 (1938): 467–489, here 467.
59. Helene Deutsch, "Some Forms of Emotional Disturbance and Their Relationship To Schizophrenia," *Psychoanalytic Quarterly* 11 (1942): 301–321.
60. Robert P. Knight, "Borderline States," *Bulletin of the Menninger Clinic* 17 (1953): 1–12.
61. Otto Kernberg, "Borderline Personality Organization," *Journal of the American Psychoanalytic Association* 15 (1967): 641–685, here 657.
62. Otto Kernberg, "Clinical Dimensions of Masochism," *Journal of the American Psychoanalytic Association* 36 (1988): 1005–1029, here 1013.
63. E. Mansell Pattison and Joel Kahan, "The Deliberate Self-Harm Syndrome," *American Journal of Psychiatry* 140 (1983): 867–72.
64. Ibid., 867.
65. Joel Kahan and E. Mansell Pattison, "Proposal for a Distinctive Diagnosis: The Deliberate Self-Harm Syndrome (DSH)," *Suicide and Life-Threatening Behavior* 14 (1984): 17–35.
66. See Ruth Leys, *Trauma: A Genealogy* (Chicago: University of Chicago Press, 2000).
67. Victoria Lewin-Fetter, "Self-harm on Either Side of the Pond," *The Lancet* 376, no. 9748 (2010): 1224.
68. Elizabeth Grosz, *Volatile Bodies: Toward a Corporeal Feminism* (Bloomington: Indiana University Press, 1994), here 141.
69. Grosz, 142.
70. Grosz.
71. Jane Kilby, "Carved in Skin: Bearing Witness to Self Harm," *Thinking Through the Skin*, eds., Sara Ahmed and Jackie Stacey (London: Routledge, 2001), 124–42, here 126.
72. Kay Inckle, *Writing on the Body? Thinking Through Gendered. Embodiment and Marked Flesh* (Newcastle: Cambridge Scholars, 2007), xi.
73. American Psychiatric Association, *Diagnostic and Statistical Manual of Mental Disorders, Fifth Edition* (Arlington, VA.: American Psychiatric Association, 2013), 803. The full criteria for the disorder appears on 803–806.
74. German E. Berrios, *The History of Mental Symptoms* (Cambridge: Cambridge University Press, 1996), 444.
75. Ian Hacking, "Lost in the Forest," *London Review of Books* 35, 15 (8 August 2013): 7–8, here 8.
76. Carlos Strenger, *The Designed Self: Psychoanalysis and Contemporary Identities* (Hillsdale, NJ: The Analytic Press, 2005).

Questions

Are the classifications of mental illness stable over time?

How does the study of medical history enable us to understand our own classifications of mental illness?

Define "cutting."

Is tattooing a sign of mental illness? When and where was it considered to be such a symptom?

Why are classifications of illness such as the DSM-5 or the International Classification of Diseases (ICD) important?

Case Eight

Genes and Race

Problems: With the importance of genetics in understanding illness, why and how has the older concept of "race" reappeared in the health sciences as a category of genetic explanation? What happens when this new genetics of race is mobilized for political as well as scientific purposes?

Race in the Contemporary World

Contemporary genetics has reanimated the concept of race as a category in medical science. The ongoing debates about the relationship of older and contemporary uses of race to those in our age focus on what seems to be recycled material/arguments from some of the debates of the first "age of racial biology" in the late nineteenth century. The University of California geneticist Neil Risch stated recently that numerous studies over past decades have documented biological differences among the races with regard to susceptibility and natural history of chronic diseases, yet he asks at the same time:

> What is your definition of races? If you define it a certain way, maybe that's a valid statement. There is obviously still disagreement. . . . Scientists always disagree! A lot of the problem is terminology. I'm not even sure what race means, people use it in many different ways . . . but that doesn't preclude you from using it or the fact that it has utility.[1]

Yet this leaves open the ambiguity of race in contemporary genetics, not only in its appropriation in the public sphere but also within science.

The concept of race has remained contested in genetics to no little degree because it takes on truly different meanings in different cultural settings, irrespective of the science to which it makes reference. "Racial formation" or "racialization" comes to be an alternative manner of analyzing race as a pseudo-biological concept determined by the political intent of its users and as a historically contingent category of essential difference. "The meaning of race," as Michael Omi and Howard Winant suggested over twenty years ago, "is defined and contested in both collective action and personal practice."[2] In the process, they argue, "racial categories themselves are formed, transformed, destroyed and re-formed."[3] Racial formation, then, refers to the process of investing meaning in racial categories—"the extension of racial meaning to relationships, social practices, or groups" previously understood in nonracial terms.[4] Thus the very absence or presence of the concept reflects absolute boundaries of biologically fixed groups whose character is as radically circumscribed as its biology. The contingent nature of such categories are seen or not seen based on how a context (historical, social, cultural, including the health sciences) uses or ignores race.

David Theo Goldberg argued recently that in contemporary Western neoliberalism there is a silencing of race as a long-term process, embedded in the gradual demise of scientific racism and the associated explicitly biological theories of race.[5] Race becomes unspoken because it is no longer seen as grounded in science. But it really matters which group is the litmus test for "race." Peter Wade countered Goldberg in that he argues that Goldberg's approach privileges an overly institutional presence for race and thus loses sight of the real and continuing presence of race in contemporary societies, especially notable in biotechnological and genomic contexts. For him race is not about biology, but about a constant movement between nature and culture, mediated by classifications of Others, based on histories of Western colonialism and postcolonialism, even within the cutting edge science of race. Wade goes on to argue that, in Latin America, *racialized* difference is, if anything, made more explicit in the context of what Charles Hale has labeled "neoliberal multiculturalism."[6]

Race itself has a complex history that clearly antedates the rise of modern genetics. The *Oxford English Dictionary* traces its meaning ("a tribe, nation, or people, regarded as of common stock. In early use frequently with modifying adjective, as British race, Roman race") from, in 1572, "The Englishe race ouerrunne and daily spoiled" to a "group of several tribes or peoples, regarded as forming a distinct ethnic set" in 1612, where race is associated with color as an index of racial biology: "He is a white man and of the Race of the Tartares." By 1775, modern science takes over, and the German researcher J. F. Blumenbach and his *De Generis Humani Varietati Nativa* is cited as using race as a "more or less formal systems of classification: any of the major groupings of mankind, having in common distinct physical features or having a similar ethnic background." In 1795, the *OED* notes the popular acceptance of this view: "These Tartar tribes, which he supposes to be of the Red Race, distinct from the European White Race." Race in its modern, non-metaphoric sense has become a reflex of the *science* of biology and is not merely pseudo-science. For science and its popular reception is dynamic, changing its claims over time as to its facts. It was Wilhelm Johannsen (1857–1927) who first coined the word "gene" in 1909, well after race had become an acceptable concept within the health sciences of the day.

By the close of the nineteenth century, certain ideas about the science of race became commonplaces: there was always a fixed boundary, a bright line, between races; there was a hierarchy of the races based on observable phenomena; mixed races were inherently inferior to pure races; race was mapped in some inherent way onto geography; that less able races could trump superior races by sheer numbers. Now all of these claims were clothed in the newest sciences of the day, from epidemiology and its statistical apparatus to eugenics and early genetics with its models of inheritance to clinical medicine with its classification of diseases and its claims of a biological and often inherent etiology for such diseases.

Yet it is clear that in using the science of race everything is political, and all science, as objective as it may wish to be, grapples with the political use and implications of its claims. Here we can turn to Mitchell Ash, who proposes that historians and sociologists of science adopt a dynamic view of the relationship between science and politics in which each serves as a resource for the other. Science may serve as a "cognitive, rhetorical or institutional resource," and it also transforms the very content or practice of science in that political context.[7] Even the origins of modern genetics reflect this. If we move from the rediscovery in 1900 of Gregor Mendel's 1866 and 1868 description of the patterns of inheritance in sweet peas (*Pisum sativum*) by three European botanists, Hugo de Vries, Carl Correns, and Erich von Tschermak, we can note the beginnings of the politicization of the claims of this new science. Sheila Faith Weiss notes that

> German eugenics incorporated genetics into its racial argument as early as 1913 when Eugen Fischer published his study of the so-called Rehobother Bastards—an investigation of the biological effects of racial intermarriage between Dutch settlers and native Hottentots in German Southwest Africa—published in 1913. Fischer's study was billed as the first successful demonstration of Mendelism in a human population, although that claim has been recently and rightfully called into question.[8]

In the United States as Kenneth Ludmerer notes, geneticists' enthusiasm for eugenics during the period 1905–1915 was modified in the American context.[9] Non-scientists highly politicized the question of eugenics and inheritance, such as in the law drafted by Harry Laughlin (1880–1943). This was adopted by the Commonwealth of Virginia to authorize the sterilization of those deemed to be socially "inferior." This was later adopted into the Nazi Law for Protection Against Genetically Defective Offspring in 1933 that provided the legal basis for sterilizations in Germany. It was Laughlin's law that called forth Oliver Wendell Holmes, Jr.'s comment in "Buck vs. Bell" that:

> We have seen more than once that the public welfare may call upon the best citizens for their lives. It would be strange if it could not call upon those who already sap the strength of the State for these lesser sacrifices, often not felt to be such by those concerned, in order to prevent our being swamped with incompetence. It is better for all the world, if instead of waiting to execute degenerate offspring for crime, or to let them starve for their imbecility, society can prevent those who are manifestly unfit from continuing their kind. The principle that sustains compulsory vaccination is broad enough to cover cutting the Fallopian tubes. Three generations of imbeciles are enough.

Yet American geneticists withdrew their support between 1915 and 1924 to such application of their science, but as Ludmerer notes, that they did not "publically condemn eugenics."[10]

Our "second age of biology" seems to be repeating some of these claims (albeit with substantially different evidence) of the first. The medical concept of race as studied in the medical humanities is a contested and complex notion with histories that reflect the complexity of the idea of science in various cultures and with various national trajectories.

The litmus test for race science in nineteenth-century Europe was the Jews, defined as a homogenous racial cohort rather than as a religion. In the United States, it was the African American. The nineteenth-century practice of labeling both groups as a "degenerate" race was a means of labeling them as inferior within the terms of nineteenth-century scientific racism. But the idea of a bright line of race distinguished the Jews of Western Europe, who were gradually being integrated into civil society during the course of the nineteenth century. As more and more of the external signs of differences—the liberation from the ghetto, the linguistic integration into European culture and language, the increased social and professional mobility of Jews, the abandonment of required or traditional dress, the reform of religious practices—made the Jew invisible, inherent racial characteristics were discovered that marked Jewish biological difference. A racially defined Jew was one whose body betrayed itself. Thus William-Frédéric Edwards, a physician, argued in 1829 that races remained constant all over the world.[11] Edwards's proof for this was the stability of the Jews all over the world.[12] Edwards's friend the Scottish physician Robert Knox brought as proof the "fact" that the portraits of Jews in Egyptian tombs resembled the Jews of contemporary London![13] Oscar Wilde was, of course, right decades later when he argued that nature copies art rather than art copying nature. The reality of the world mirrored the fantasies of its observers as Karen Barad notes, for we are "responsible for the world of which we are a part, not because it is an arbitrary construction of our choosing but because reality is sedimented out of particular practices that we have a role in shaping and through which we are shaped."[14] The fantasies about the Jewish body demanded such arguments of continuity. In 1841 Hubert Lauvergne, a follower of the phrenologist Franz Joseph Gall, argued that contemporary Greeks bore the proud face and skull of ancient Greece, while the "immutability of the Jewish type" proved their degeneracy.[15]

Race and Jewish Genes in Contemporary Germany

In 2010, a scandal rocked Germany that illustrated how very much the debate about "racial biology" is alive—but is articulated quite differently in terms of its location and politics—in the early twenty-first century. Thilo Sarrazin, then a prominent member of the SPD, former senator of finance for the State of Berlin from 2002 until 2009 and in the fall of 2010 a well-respected member of the Executive Board of the *Deutsche Bundesbank*, published a best-selling screed, *Deutschland Schafft Sich Ab* ("Germany Does Away With Itself"), against German multiculturalism in August 2010. In it he decried the dilution of "German" society by the reproductive capacity of a permanent and unassimilatable underclass of "Muslim immigrants" in Germany.[16] Yet it was his comment that "all Jews share a particular gene" that "makes them different from other peoples" which caused an international uproar.[17] (And forced his resignation from the *Deutsche Bundesbank* in September 2010.) This claim became the focus of much of the German as well as international engagement with Sarrazin. It was most crudely articulated in an interview with *Welt am Sonntag* following the publication of his book in which he stated that "all Jews share a certain gene as all Basques share a certain gene that distinguishes these from other people."[18] Race, a concept so fraught with its historical association with Nazi biology and patterns of extermination, was virtually inexpressible in Germany.

In his book, Sarrazin also clumsily links his argument about the danger of "Muslim immigrants" to the German nation by writing about the "average higher intelligence of the Jews" passed through a Jewish gene. He thus sought to escape the charge of racism by praising the "race" of the Jews, a telling gesture of philo-Semitism with a long history, as the German Jewish columnist and gadfly Henryk Broder was quick to point out.[19] This recycling of nineteenth-century claims of Jewish particularism struck a deep chord. Ironically his "praise" of Jewish superiority seemed to overshadow the substance of his attack on the "Muslim immigrants" in Germany. In Germany, this notion of a Jewish genetic identity was read as a clearly political statement about discredited notions of race: "Whoever tries to define Jews by their genetic makeup, even when it is superficially positive in tone, is in the grip of a race mania that Jews do not share," said Stephan Kramer, secretary general of the Central Council of Jews in Germany, quoted in the same *New York Times* article in which Sarrazin's views were cited.

Thilo Sarrazin's book belongs to a more or less recent recycling of nineteenth-century claims about the self-imposed nature of an explicit Jewish biological (read: racial) "difference." Sometimes this bright line of racial difference is framed not as a deficit but as an advantage; Jews as a collective are, for example, smarter than other peoples. But it is the very notion of a biological collective, of a "race" defined by biology and perpetuated by a group strategy ("conspiracy" in nineteenth-century anti-Semitic parlance) that is a problem. And, to be accurate, the supposed advantage is often revealed to be a true disadvantage to the society as a whole (and even to the so-called Jewish genetic collective itself).

The creation of a "genetic cohort" as a homogenous collective in the same sense that "race" had been used to unify and level groups in nineteenth-century science is a ghost in the machine of modern genetics.[20] Lynn B. Jorde and Stephen P. Wooding noted,

> New genetic data has enabled scientists to re-examine the relationship between human genetic variation and "race." . . . These [genetic] clusters are also correlated with some traditional concepts of race, but the correlations are imperfect because genetic variation tends to be distributed in a continuous, overlapping fashion among populations. Therefore, ancestry, or even race, may in some cases prove useful in the biomedical

> setting, but direct assessment of disease-related genetic variation will ultimately yield more accurate and beneficial information."[21]

Francis Collins, head of the American Human Genome Project, does care:

> The downside of using race, whether in research or in the practice of medicine is that we are reifying it as if it has more biological significance than it deserves. Race is an imperfect surrogate for the causative information we seek. To the extent that we continue to use it, we are suggesting to the rest of the world that it is very reliable and that racial categories have more biological meaning than they do. We may even appear to suggest something that I know is not true: that there are bright lines between populations and that races are biologically distinct.[22]

The "bright lines" that absolutely define complex and heterogeneous cohorts by using highly contested forms of evidence such as "intelligence" are to be avoided in any modern reading of genetics.

The genetics that claims that there is a "gene" for "the Jews" (at least for the Jewish priestly class), the Cohen Modal Haplotype (CMH), remains in doubt.[23] The scientists who claimed a Cohen Modal Haplotype were recently forced to redo their study and just recently refuted their own claim, acknowledging that there is no such thing. Indeed, recent work argues the contrary, that at least the Ashkenazi Jewish population (European Jews) is genetically more diverse than other people of European descent, despite previous assumptions that Ashkenazi Jews have been an isolated population.[24] Researchers looked for close to one million single nucleotide polymorphisms (SNPs): common alternative spellings in the genome, analogous to American and British spellings of words such as organize/organise. One measure of genetic diversity in a population is heterozygosity, or how many of the SNPs inherited from the mother and father are different; a more inbred population has less heterozygosity. "We were surprised to find evidence that Ashkenazi Jews have higher heterozygosity than Europeans, contradicting the widely-held presumption that they have been a largely isolated group," said first author Dr. Steven Bray. Other fields have been less willing or able to reject such reductive genetic models. As a recent study of the sociology of race noted:

> One respondent, who was involved in studies on Jewish populations, mentioned that his research was likely to be misinterpreted and misused by some, but insisted that it was out of his hands. He said that people used to approach him and ask whether it could be "genetically" tested if they were Jewish. He was adamant to stress that being

> Jewish was not about genetics and it was wrong that this research was interpreted this way, but claimed that he had no control over these types of "popular" representations of his work.[25]

And Sarrazin very much falls into this category of a popular misuse of (in his case) very, very bad science.

In twenty-first-century Germany can the Jews still be defined a "race" historically? If they are, as Sarrazin shows, this can be read as having positive rather than negative connotations, as it seems to be an attempt at a politically correct statement, at least in Sarrazin's eyes. It comes to be a so-called philo-Semitic argument that is still rooted however in the notion of a homogenous Jewish genetic (read: racial) type. For the first age of biology, for the nineteenth century, the Jew defined racial, and that meant biological difference. And all Jews were equivalent. Hidden within the modern, acculturated body of the nineteenth-century European Jew is a racially defined Jew whose body betrays itself as different.

Smart Jews in the Historical Debates about Race

The "Jewish type" in the nineteenth century was often defined by one salient quality, that of a Jewish intelligence or cleverness. This is the claim that Sarrazin's book makes in its discussion of Jewish "higher intelligence" as created by Jewish marrying practices.[26] This nineteenth-century view has a peculiar continuity after the Holocaust. In 1969, Ernest van den Haag presented a similar (non-Jewish) reading of "Jewish intellectual superiority."[27] The biologist van den Haag suggested that Jewish males of higher intelligence were encouraged to reproduce and "literally for millennia, the brightest had the best chance to marry and produce children, and their children had the best chance to survive infancy."[28] Van den Haag also argued that Christians sacrificed their "good" genes by making their priests celibate; the Jews rewarded smart rabbis with the best wives and the most support for the families. Christian genes for intelligence were diminished, and genes for Jewish superior intelligence were reinforced.

> The church offered the only career in which intellectual ability was rewarded, regardless of the origin of its bearer. . . . But the priesthood exacted a price: celibacy. Which meant that the most intelligent portion of the population did not have offspring; their genes were siphoned off, generation after generation, into the church, and not returned to the world's, or even the church's, genetic supply.[29]

This is the reduction of all "Jewish" experience to a single model of genetic transmission that enabled van den Haag's argument to work.

Van den Haag's view is a "scientific" formulation of the views espoused by individuals such as the Jewish mathematician Norbert Wiener and his friend the Marxist mathematical geneticist J. B. S. Haldane and which the American Jewish sociologist Lewis S. Feuer comes to call the "Wiener/Haldane" thesis.[30] According to Wiener: "The biological habits of the Christians tended to breed out of the race whatever hereditary qualities make for learning where as the biological habits of the Jew tended to breed these qualities in."[31] Feuer noted the error in this logic, pointing to a long history of anxiety about misalliances among Jewish families.[32] Few rich parents sought out poor scholars, they sought out equivalent marriages either with wealthy Jews or with the scions of established rabbinic families. The range of marriage structures among Jews in Europe was also altered by the Enlightenment and by the rise of the women's movement in Central Europe in the late nineteenth century. It is the reduction of all "Jewish" experience to a single model of genetic transmission that enabled van den Haag's argument to work.

The van den Haag argument stresses that Jewish isolation and social pariah-dom had a positive biological outcome—it enabled Jews to maintain their superior intelligence, as they were not accountable to forms of social and cultural pressure that "deformed" the intelligence of the Christian cohort. Richard J. Herrnstein and Charles Murray's best selling book of 1994, *The Bell Curve: Intelligence and Class Structure in American Life,* drew attention to the debate about the relationship between inheritance and intelligence, a debate which in the American context is read as a comment on "race" (read: blackness) and lower intelligence rather than in Sarrazin's text as "Muslim immigrants" and lower intelligence.[33] Sarrazin cites the discussion of the *Bell Curve* early in his book[34] as one of his proofs not only for the superiority of the Jews but also, by extension, of his general argument about the dangers of a biologically inferior underclass, in his case the "Muslim immigrants" rather than African Americans. There is no question that *The Bell Curve* was in the 1990s (and evidently still is) read as a book of race and intelligence. In *The Bell Curve,* intelligence becomes a discussion of character and virtue. While this debate about the relationship between "race" and "IQ" has been sporadically carried out over the past three decades around the work of Arthur Robert Jensen, William Shockley, and J. Philippe Rushton, little attention has been paid to the ethical and moral questions that adumbrate these studies.[35] Herrnstein and Murray's presentation in this regard is neither the most extensive nor the most hotly contested. Even though it deals with "cognitive class" and not explicitly with race as defined by skin color, it repeats the collateral question addressed by much of the earlier literature of this topic. Virtue and morality are the real objects of *The Bell Curve*—and these qualities are posited positively or negatively at both ends of the curve.

For there are two ends to Herrnstein and Murray's "bell curve," each of them thin and rare. As rare as is the lowest end of the curve, those of lowest intelligence, according to the classic argument, it is equally true that the upper end of the curve is also rare. It is fascinating that little or no attention is given in the analysis of such studies to the "normal" center. The thin ends define the problem—the "normal" center is understood as the model of intelligence and therefore also the model of virtue. It is erroneously assumed in these investigations that only the deviant, following the model of the pathological in medicine, can provide insight into the normal. And thus the center—the two standard deviations from the norm in this model—is invisible. It remains the implicit site of virtue though (or because) of its "average" intelligence.

Given the American political climate of the mid-1990s, one can understand why the Herrnstein and Murray book has attracted much attention in its evocation of the myth of a permanent underclass (read: of African Americans) whose high rate of reproduction, low intelligence, and degenerate sociopathic genes have led to an America where it is dangerous to walk the streets of the big cities. Or as Herrnstein and Murray note, "high intelligence also provides some protection against lapsing into criminality for people who otherwise are at risk."[36] According to this model, criminals are dumb and dumb people are criminals. This ahistorical reconstruction ignores all of the complex reading of the relationship between "intelligence" (however that is defined) and "crime" (however that is defined).[37] According to contemporaries, New York's Hell's Kitchen in the 1860s was full of atavistic Irishmen who made the streets unsafe. They too were literally seen as a race apart and were accused of reproducing at an uncomfortably high rate. The racial sign of their lower intelligence could be seen in their simian brow and saddle nose! Such myths about the relationship of "low intelligence" and "race" are stock ones in the repertory of Western science from at least the mid-eighteenth century. They function to dispel the anxiety of an established society about the source of social instability. Identify your potential enemy and you can control your anxiety! Thus the focus on the lower end of the bell curve has been an attempt to locate the origins of the anxiety about individual risk in a stereotyped category.

But what about those who are too smart? Little attention has been paid to the other end of the spectrum, to the thin line at the other end of the so-called bell curve. It is this end that serves as a prophylaxis against crime. Herrnstein and Murray devote only one page to the highest group in terms of intelligence—"Ashkenasic Jews of European origins" who "test higher than any other ethnic group." Based on this model that equates intelligence with virtue, we would come to expect that the higher the intelligence, the greater the protection against criminality, the greater the virtue of the group. According to Herrnstein and Murray, "Jews in America and Britain have an overall IQ mean somewhere between a half and a full standard deviation above the mean, with the source of the difference concentrated in the verbal component."[38] Such test scores, however, are not sufficient for them to establish the superior intelligence of the Jews; they also rely on "analyses of occupational and scientific attainment by Jews, which constantly show their disproportionate level of success, usually by orders of magnitude, in various inventories of scientific and artistic achievement." But it is equally important to understand that the implication of such studies is the identification and quantifiability of virtue, and that such rather crude types of analogies are just as likely to draw the virtue of the Jews into question as to posit them as the cite of virtue. Such arguments are variants on the myths that attribute superior intelligence to the Jews as a cohort.

Sarrazin's Primary Source

Most recently the claim of a Jewish superior intelligence has been espoused by Sarrazin's major but highly derivative source for the "science of race," the self-described "evolutionary psychologist and . . . research[er] into Jewish-gentile relations," Kevin MacDonald, the author of a trilogy on Jewish reproductive strategies.[39] MacDonald is professor of psychology at California State University-Long Beach, Long Beach. Despite the highly derivative nature of his work, to quote MacDonald:

> As indicated by the summaries of my books, my training as an evolutionist as well as the evidence compiled by historians leads me to conceptualize Judaism as self-interested groups whose interests often conflict with segments of the gentile community. Anti-Jewish attitudes and behavior have been a pervasive feature of the Jewish experience since the beginnings of the Diaspora well over 2000 years ago.[40]

For MacDonald Judaism is less a religion than a biological strategy:

> The basic proposal is that Judaism can be interpreted as a set of ideological structures and behaviors that have resulted in the following features: (1) the segregation of the Jewish gene pool from surrounding gentile societies; (2) resource and reproductive competition with gentile host societies; (3) high levels of within-group cooperation and altruism among Jews; and (4) eugenic efforts directed at producing high intelligence, high investment parenting, and commitment to group, rather than individual, goals.[41]

And that more over "that intellectual defenses of Judaism and of Jewish theories of anti-Semitism have throughout its history played a critical role in maintaining Judaism as a group evolutionary strategy." Sarrazin paraphrases the latter[42] by stating that the idea of intelligence was a scientific discovery by the Hamburg psychologist Wilhelm Stern, who was forced to flee Nazi Germany because of his Jewish backgrounds. Firstly, this is not at all an accurate representation of the modern history of intelligence and intelligence testing, which begins in France and has its own American development. Secondly, Sarrazin calls upon Stern as a Jewish scientist as a means of arguing, as does MacDonald, that the very idea of intelligence is a Jewish invention and therefore beyond any accusation of anti-Semitism, as the intelligence of the Jewish scientist is a sign of Jewish genetic advantage. But that advantage is itself proof of a Jewish genetic conspiracy. MacDonald's views are rather pure nineteenth-century biological anti-Semitism now cloaked in the rhetoric of an evolutionary biology driven by simplistic genetic models. Such evolutionary and genetic "just-so-stories" depend greatly on the definition of their components; science is, as has been recently remarked, always based on just-so-stories—but competent (not "good") science tests and retests its terms and assumptions so that it is dynamic in its processes and claims. MacDonald's work, like that of his predecessors, does not meet this test.

The problem with evoking such earlier racial models in the name of evolutionary biology is that it places you in odd political company. Thus MacDonald's self-descriptions quoted above begin his testimony given on Monday, January 31, 2000, as the sole "scientific" witness speaking for David Irving in the notorious trial "Irving v Penguin Books Ltd and Deborah Lipstadt" in which Irving accused the American historian Deborah Lipstadt of libeling him by labeling him a "Holocaust denier" in her 1993 *Denying the Holocaust.* To quote Justice Gray's summary:

> Irving has for his own ideological reasons persistently and deliberately misrepresented and manipulated historical evidence; that for the

> same reasons he has portrayed Hitler in an unwarrantedly favourable light, principally in relation to his attitude towards and responsibility for the treatment of the Jews; that he is an active Holocaust denier; that he is anti-Semitic and racist, and that he associates with right-wing extremists who promote neo-Nazism.[43]

The upshot of the trial was that Irving and by extension, MacDonald, were declared by the British court to be anti-Semites. This can certainly be noted in MacDonald's response on a blog devoted to "white identity, interests, and culture" to the recent critiques of Sarrazin by noting, "No need to discuss the fact that Jewish genetic commonality discovered by (Jewish) population geneticists can only be explained ultimately by the fact that the Jews have always had a race mania."[44] The very notion that the Jews have a "mania" seems to locate Jewish intelligence in the realm of the pathological.

Smart Genes; Smart Jews

The notion that there is a Jewish genetic identity did not end with the dismissal of MacDonald's "evidence" in a court of law. It has reappeared in other more recent forms. In 2006, Gregory Cochran, Jason Hardy, and Henry Harpending—all anthropologists at the University of Utah—made quite a splash with a published study suggesting that Jewish "superior" intelligence was the result of selective "in-breeding." Their paper, "Natural History of Ashkenazi Intelligence," argued that Jewish intelligence is simply a compensatory genetic error linked to other "Jewish" genetic diseases, like Tay-Sachs, Gaucher's Disease, or Fanconi's anemia. As the authors write: "perhaps most of the characteristic Ashkenazi genetic diseases fall into this category. Selection has imposed a heavy human cost: not crippling at the population level, cheaper than the malaria-defense mutations like sickle cell and G6PD deficiency, but tragic nonetheless."[45] This is an elaboration of the biological claims espoused by MacDonald. Every brilliant Jew is simultaneously a frail Jew, living the life of the mind rather than that of the body.

The Columbia University geneticist Robert Pollack is much more dismissive of this claim of specific genetic qualities that define abstractions such as intelligence:

> But all characteristics of a person that we perceive to be interesting—like intelligence, kindness, musical ability, obnoxiousness—to the extent that these have a genetic component, it will be contained in thousands or perhaps tens of thousands of genes. We have no capacity at present to measure that.

Race is not the equivalent to a genetic cohort, and ephemeral qualities such as "intelligence" are poor proof of genetic transmission. Rather Pollack argues (as quoted and paraphrased in a *Jerusalem Post* article by Abraham Rabinovich):

> The astonishing flowering of Jewish genius and accomplishment in the present century... may prove to be an autumnal exuberance of color that will be followed by a long, pallid winter in which Jews, 50 years hence, will be no more accomplished than anyone else. The Yiddish phrase, "A Yid miz zich mitchen" ("A Jew has to struggle"), used to be a wry, if obvious, comment on the Jewish condition. In retrospect, the phrase can be seen as the secret formula for Jewish success.[46]

Thilo Sarrazin's work is a rehash of older, highly discredited versions of a homogenous Jewish biological identity proven by a higher Jewish IQ. As with earlier versions of such claims, the "Jews" are always played off against some other groups that are seen as less successful biologically. But of course, as with Sarrazin's view as well as in the claims of his sources, intelligence is measured by social accomplishment—a faulty measure, as a genetic "cause" assumes a constant rate of accomplishment, and accomplishment changes its meaning over time. Such argument about Jewish intelligence rests on individual accomplishments—such as Nobel Prizes and violin virtuosi—of those who are labeled or self-identified as "Jews," and these individual accomplishments may well be a reflex of a culture of learning and performance by individuals placed in a specific Diaspora situation. As Albert Einstein pointed out in 1929: "If my theory of relativity is proven successful, Germany will claim me as a German and France will declare that I am a citizen of the world. Should my theory prove untrue, France will say that I am a German and Germany will declare that I am a Jew."[47] Categories, Einstein implies, are created by contexts.

Being "Jewish" was only one identity for Einstein, if an important one. He never made the same claim about his rather amateurish but passionate violin playing eliciting the envy of nations. Such categories as "Jewish Nobel Prize winners" are used to chronicle accomplishment of individuals, especially at moments when the social situation permits these individuals to excel and a group needs to identify with these accomplishments to answer charges of inherent difference and assumed inferiority. When in 2011 Daniel Shechtman of the Technion-Israel Institute of Technology in Haifa won the Nobel Prize for Chemistry, there was a great deal of interest in Israel about the fact that "Israel has an impressive showing when it comes to Nobel winners, with 10 laureates in its 63-year history."[48] Not *Jewish* Nobel Prize winners but *Israeli*, for all of the reasons noted above.

Such claims about intelligence decline as the pressure to excel in any identifiable group diminishes and the group ceases to need "heroes." If this were not the case, the recent, rapid decrease in the number of self-identified Jews who are applying to American medical schools could mean that Jews may have lost God's grace—but perhaps are also becoming less "diseased" or more at risk for criminality as their intelligence declines. Actually, what has happened in the United States is that self-identified Jews are fitting more closely into the profile of the American middle class! They are making choices about their professions based on their middle-class identity rather than the desires of their parents. And the "New Jews"—the Asian Americans, an equally invented category—are filling the medical schools because of the social pressures that define this as a major route of success in the American Diaspora.

For Sarrazin, it is the anxiety about the "Muslim immigrants" that shapes his argument about the Jews. "Germany destroys itself" is the title of his book. It is in line with a long history of seeing the decay of the present in the light of an edenic, prelapsarian (or here pre-Holocaust) past. The irony is that it is quite possible that the next generation of German geniuses may be members of perceived marginal groups, as the Jews were in the nineteenth century. The sad thing is that Sarrazin uses in a German setting the Jews as his most successful case, marking perhaps a moment where the Holocaust (except among German Jews) no longer plays a role in the consciousness of minority questions. For if Sarrazin's "Muslim immigrants" are too stupid to be citizens, the Nazi's Jews were far too clever to remain citizens. What goes around comes around.

Notes

1. Neal Risch, "The whole side of it—an interview with Neil Risch by Jane Gitschier," *PLoS Genetics* 1, no. 1 (July 2005): e14.
2. Michael Omi and Howard Winant, *Racial Formation in the United States from the 1960s to the 1980s* (New York: Routledge, 1986), 61.
3. Ibid., 61.
4. Ibid., 64.
5. David Theo Goldberg, *The Threat of Race: Reflections on Racial Neoliberalism* (Oxford and Malden, MA: Wiley-Blackwell, 2009).
6. Peter Wade, "The Presence and Absence of Race," *Patterns of Prejudice* 44 (2010): 43–60.

7. Mitchell Ash, "Wissenschaft und Politik als Ressourcen für einander," in Rüdiger vom Buch and Brigitte Kaderas, eds., *Wissenschaften und Wissenschaftspolitik. Bestandsaufnahme und Perspektiven der Forschung* (Stuttgart: Franz Steiner, 2002), 32–49.
8. Sheila Faith Weiss, "Human Genetics and Politics as Mutually Beneficial Resources: The Case of the Kaiser Wilhelm Institute for Anthropology, Human Heredity and Eugenics During the Third Reich," *Journal of the History of Biology* (2006) 39: 41–88.
9. Kenneth Ludmerer, "American Geneticists and the Eugenics Movement, 1905–1935," *Journal of the History of Biology*, 2 (1969): 337–362.
10. Ibid., 352.
11. All citations from Martin S. Staum, *Labeling People: French Scholars on Society, Race, and Empire 1815–1848* (Montreal and Kingston: McGill-Queens University Press, 2003).
12. Edwards quoted in Staum, 129.
13. Staum, 130.
14. Karen Barad, *Meeting the Universe Halfway: Quantum Physics and the Entanglement of Matter and Meaning* (Duke University Press Books, 2007), 390.
15. Ibid., 59.
16. Thilo Sarrazin, *Deutschland schafft sich ab: Wie wir unser Land aufs Spiel setzen* (München: Deutsche Verlags-Anstalt, 2010), here 95.
17. Judy Dempsey, "Comments by German on Minorities Are Criticized," *The New York Times*, August 29, 2010.
18. "Gibt es auch eine genetische Identität?" "Alle Juden teilen ein bestimmtes Gen, Basken haben bestimmte Gene, die sie von anderen unterscheiden." Andrea Seibel, Hajo Schumacher, Joachim Fahrun, "'Ich bin kein Rassist'; Thilo Sarrazin, Bundesbank-Vorstand und früherer Berliner Finanzsenator, über seine These, muslimische Migranten hätten größere Probleme als andere Einwanderer," *Welt am Sonntag*, August 29, 2010, 4. See also Stephen Lowman, "German Politician Stirs Controversy with His Inflammatory Views on Muslims and Jews," *The Washington Post*, August 31, 2010, and Michael Woodhead, "'All Jews Share a Certain Gene': German Banker Sparks Outrage with 'Stupid' Comments," *The Daily Mail*, August 30, 2010. Sarrazin does not see any problem with these earlier remarks, as he recently stated in an interview: "Sarrazin: ... aber ich hatte mich so viel mit genetischen Fragen beschäftigt, dass ich die Sache gar nicht als dermaßen explosiv verstand, wie sie sich dann herausstellte. Welt Online: Sonst nichts? Sarrazin: Nein. Ich habe mir die kritischen Passagen öfter angesehen und nichts Falsches oder Anstößiges gefunden." *Die Welt-on-line*, January 28, 2012, http://www.welt.de/politik/deutschland/article13805710/Thilo-Sarrazin-geisselt-die-Wut-der-Pharisaeer.html (accessed January 19, 2012).
19. "Der Publizist und Autor Henryk M.Broder äußert sich zur Debatte um Thilo Sarrazin. Auszüge aus einem Interview mit SPIEGEL TV," *Der Spiegel*, September 7, 2010, http://www.spiegel.de/video/video-1082930.html (accessed December 1, 2013).
20. Susan Oyama, *Evolution's Eye: A Systems View of the Biology-Culture Divide* (Durham, NC: Duke University Press, 2000).
21. Lynn B. Jorde and Stephen P. Wooding, "Genetic Variation, Classification and 'Race,'" *Nature Genetics* 36 (2004): S28 - S33.
22. Anon., *The Economist*, April 12, 2006: 80.

23. Michael F. Hammer, Doron M. Behar, Tatiana M. Karafet, Fernando L. Mendez, Brian Hallmark, Tamar Erez, Lev A. Zhivotovsky, Saharon Rosset, and Karl Skorecki, "Extended Y Chromosome Haplotypes Resolve Multiple and Unique Lineages of the Jewish Priesthood," *Human Genetics* 126 (2009): 719–24 and Anatole Klyosov, "Comment on the paper: Extended Y Chromosome Haplotypes Resolve Multiple and Unique Lineages of the Jewish Priesthood," *Human Genetics* 126 (2009): 719–724. But see also: Michael Hammer, et al., (2009b), "Response," *Human Genetics* 126 (2009): 725–726.
24. Steven M. Bray, Jennifer G. Mulle, Anne F. Dodd, Ann E. Pulver, Stephen Wooding, and Stephen T. Warren, "Signatures of Founder Effects, Admixture, and Selection in the Ashkenazi Jewish Population," *Proceedings of the National Academy of Sciences of the U S A* 107 (2010): 16222–7.
25. Yulia Egorova, "DNA evidence? The Impact of Genetic Research on Historical Debates," *BioSocieties* 5 (2010): 348–365.
26. Sarrazin, *Deutschland*, 94–95
27. Ernest van den Haag, *The Jewish Mystique*, 2nd ed. (1969; repr., New York: Stein and Day, 1977), 13–25.
28. Ibid., 14.
29. Ibid., 15.
30. Lewis S. Feuer, *Scientific Intellectual: The Psychological and Sociological Origins of Modern Science* (New York: Basic Books, 1963), 308 and more extensively in his Lewis S. Feuer, "The Sociobiological Theory of Jewish Intellectual Achievement," in Joseph B. Maier and Chaim I. Waxman, eds., *Ethnicity, Identity, and History: Essays in Memory of Werner J. Cahnman* (New Brunswick: Transaction, 1983), 93–125.
31. Norbert Wiener, *Ex-Prodigy: My Childhood and Youth* (New York: Simon and Schuster, 1953), here 11. He is evoking a conversation with Haldane that echo the views of Haldane such as expressed in the Muirhead lectures given by him at Birmingham University in February and March 1937 and printed as J. B. S. Haldane, *Heredity and Politics* (London: Allen & Unwin, 1938), relevant material 162.
32. Feuer, "Sociobiological Theory of Jewish Intellectual Achievement."
33. Richard J. Herrnstein and Charles Murray, *The Bell Curve: Intelligence and Class Structure in American Life* (New York: The Free Press, 1994). The comments on Jewish superior intelligence are to be found on 275.
34. Ibid., 96.
35. On the general questions of "race" and/or "intelligence" before and after *The Bell Curve* see Richard E. Nisbett, *Intelligence and How To Get It: Why Schools and Cultures Count* (New York: W. W. Norton, 2010); Ashley Montagu, *Race and IQ* (New York: Oxford University Press, 1999); Sander L. Gilman, *Smart Jews: The Construction of the Image of Jewish Superior Intelligence* (Lincoln: University of Nebraska Press, 1996); Joe L. Kincheloe; Shirley R. Steinberg; Aaron David Gresson, eds., *Measured Lies: The Bell Curve Examined* (New York: St. Martin's Press, 1996); Claude S. Fischer, *Inequality by Design: Cracking The Bell Curve Myth* (Princeton, NJ: Princeton University Press, 1996); Russell Jacoby; Naomi Glauberman; Richard J. Herrnstein, eds., *The Bell Curve Debate: History, Documents, Opinions* (New York: Times Books, 1995); Steve Fraser, *The Bell Curve Wars: Race, Intelligence, and the Future of America* (New York: Basic Books, 1995); Robert S. Albert, ed., *Genius and Eminence*

(Oxford: Pergamon, 1992); Roger Pearson, *Race, Intelligence and Bias in Academe* (Washington, DC: Scott-Townsend Publishers, 1991); Elaine Mensh and Harry Mensh, *The IQ Mythology: Class, Race, Gender, And Inequality* (Carbondale, IL: Southern Illinois University Press, 1991); Wilhelm Quitzow, *Intelligenz, Erbe oder Umwelt?: wissenschaftliche und politische Kontroversen seit der Jahrhundertwende* (Stuttgart: J.B. Metzler, 1990); Paul Davis Chapman, *Schools as Sorters: Lewis M. Terman, Applied Psychology, and the Intelligence Testing Movement, 1890–1930* (New York: New York University Press, 1988); Raymond E. Fancher, *The Intelligence Men: Makers of the I.Q. Controversy* (New York: Norton, 1985); R. C. Lewontin, Steven Rose and Leon J. Kamin, *Not in Our Genes: Biology, Ideology, and Human Nature* (New York: Pantheon, 1984), 83–130; Stephen Jay Gould, *The Mismeasure of Man* (New York: Norton, 1981); Michel Schiff, Richard Lewontin, et al., *Education and Class: The Irrelevance of IQ Genetic Studies* (Oxford: Clarendon Press, 1986); Brian Evans, *IQ and Mental Testing: An Unnatural Science and its Social History* (London; New York: Macmillan, 1981); David Andrew Gersh, "The Development And Use Of I.Q. Tests In the United States From 1900–1930" (Diss., State University of New York at Stony Brook. Thesis, 1981); Leon J. Kamin, *The Science and Politics of I.Q.* (Potomac, Md.: L. Erlbaum Associates; distributed by Halsted Press, New York, 1974); Thomas Pogue Weinland, "A History of the I. Q. in America, 1890–1941" (PhD diss., Columbia University, 1970).

36. Herrnstein and Murray, *The Bell Curve*, 235.
37. See Carl E. Pope, "Race and Crime Revisited," *Crime and Delinquency* 25 (1979): 347–57.
38. Herrnstein and Murray, *The Bell Curve*, 275.
39. Kevin MacDonald, *A People That Shall Dwell Alone: Judaism as a Group Evolutionary Strategy* (Westport, Conn.: Praeger, 1994); *Separation and Its Discontents: Toward an Evolutionary Theory of Anti-Semitism* (Westport, Conn.: Praeger, 1998); *The Culture of Critique: An Evolutionary Analysis of Jewish Involvement in Twentieth-Century Intellectual and Political Movements* (Westport, CT: Praeger, 1998).
40. Kevin Macdonald, "Statement of Professor Kevin Macdonald," The Campaign for Real History, http://www.fpp.co.uk/Legal/Penguin/experts/MacDonald/report1.html (accessed December 1, 2013).
41. At http://www.csulb.edu/~kmacd/irving-statementCourt.html (accessed December 1, 2013).
42. Sarrazin, *Deutschland*, 96.
43. Irving v Lipstadt (2000), Paragraph 13.167.
44. Kevin Macdonald, "Policing the Elites," *The Occidental Observer* http://theoccidentalobserver.net/tooblog/?p=3309 (accessed December 1, 2013).
45. Cochran G., Hardy J., and Harpending H., "Natural History of Ashkenazi Intelligence," *Journal of Biosocial Science* 38 (2006), 659–693.
46. Abraham Rabinovich, "Farewell to Jewish gene-ius," *The Jerusalem Post*, November 30, 1998: 6.
47. Address at the Sorbonne, Paris, possibly early December 1929, quoted in *The New York Times*, February 16, 1930. Cited at http://www.oxfordreference.com/pages/samplep-18.html (accessed December 1, 2013).
48. Asaf Shtull-Trauring, "Israel's Daniel Shechtman wins 2011 Nobel Prize in Chemistry," *Haaretz*, October 5, 2011.

Questions

How does the word "race" relate to modern genetics?

What is a "race" in the nineteenth century?

What does "race" mean in Germany today?

How does Theo Sarrazin understand the politics of race in Germany?

Are the Turks a race according to Sarrazin?

Discuss the relationship between ideas of citizenship and "race."

Case Nine

Death: The Final Case

Problems: Understanding our bodies means comprehending their finite nature. How is death represented in our contemporary world, and what are the stories that have shaped our understanding of death? How are such stories tied to our understanding of whether death is our final stage of living or a passage to another stage?

Modern Death

Let us start at the beginning, which is actually fairly close to the end, in acknowledging our collective fascination with death and dying, at least on the printed page:

> She was dead. No sleep so beautiful and calm, so free from trace of pain, so fair to look upon. She seemed a creature fresh from the hand of God, and waiting for the breath of life; not one who had lived and suffered death.
>
> Her couch was dressed with here and there some winter berries and green leaves, gathered in a spot she had been used to favour. "When I die, put near me something that has loved the light, and had the sky above it always." Those were her words.
>
> She was dead. Dear, gentle, patient, noble Nell was dead. Her little bird—a poor slight thing the pressure of a finger would have crushed—was stirring nimbly in its cage; and the strong heart of its child-mistress was mute and motionless for ever.
>
> Where were the traces of her early cares, her sufferings, and fatigues? All gone. Sorrow was dead indeed in her, but peace and perfect happiness were born; imaged in her tranquil beauty and profound repose.[1]

In 1841, Charles Dickens—himself a Victorian—imagined a world under the last of the Georgian kings in *The Old Curiosity Shop*. His heroine, Nell, after innumerable torments (torments she always experienced with patience and fortitude) at the end of her life is survived by her "little bird."

The beautiful, dead, or dying woman/child, as in Dickens, was beloved of the nineteenth century. From Little Nell to *La Dame aux camellias* in all her forms, beginning with Alexandre Dumas-fils' 1848 novel and Giuseppe Verdi's 1853 opera, she becomes the touchstone for our "modern" sense of dying and death.[2] Beautiful even in death, she fixes in complex ways our model of death in literature.[3] In his *Phaedra*, Seneca wrote: "Beauty cannot stay; / would any wise man trust so frail a thing / Then use it while you may / Time is the enemy."[4] In literature, time does not cause beauty to fade. Even the death mask of *L'Inconnue de la Seine* that graced middle-class sitting rooms at the end of the century and beyond remains always beautiful. Rainer Maria Rilke sensed this in 1910 when, in *The Notebooks of Malte Laurids Brigge*, he commented on the popular mask of the beautiful dead suicide: "The face of the young drowned woman, which they took a cast of in the morgue, because it was beautiful, because it smiled, because it smiled so deceptively, as if it knew."[5] We know that her beauty will not fade, frozen as it is in the work of art. It is the promise of perfection, of beauty, even beyond corporeal death.

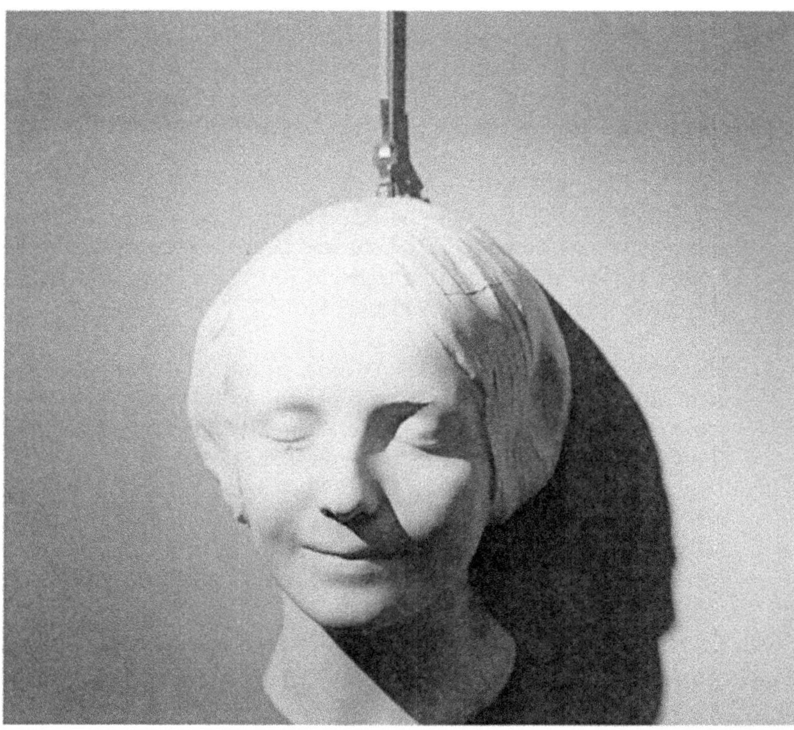

Figure 9.1. The death mask of *L'Inconnue de la Seine* (private collection).

While Victoria (1819–1901), who read Dickens's novel in 1841, found it "very interesting and cleverly written,"[6] half a century later, in 1895, Oscar Wilde found that "One would have to have a heart of stone to read the death of little Nell without dissolving into tears . . . of laughter."[7] Algernon Swinburne mocked Nell Trent as "a monster as inhuman as a baby with two heads."[8] For the moderns who no longer entertain the prospect of any beauty associated with death, who no longer see resurrection as a possibility, death has simply died. In his controversial essay of 1899, the Anglo-Jewish ethnologist Joseph Jacobs commented anonymously on "The Dying of Death":

> Death as a motive is moribund. Perhaps the most distinctive note of the modern spirit is the practical disappearance of the thought of death as an influence direct bearing on practical life. We insure our lives, it is true, but having done so think no more of the matter, except in the spirit of Wilkins Micawber when he signed a promissory note. There are no skeletons at our feasts nowadays, or at worst, they are living ones. Death has lost its terrors. . . . [9]

But not its presence.

Although the late Victorians and Edwardians—the first of the moderns—saw such beautiful representations of death as "inept and vulgarly sentimental" (quoting Aldous Huxley's reading of Little Nell in 1930), they simply do not vanish from the literary canon.[10] Today, beautiful deaths continue to be the stuff of mass culture, as when Erich Segal has Jennifer Cavilleri, the Little Nell archetype in his *Love Story* (1970), die of leukemia. Her lover, Oliver Barrett IV, mourns her before the very opening of the novel: "What can you say about a twenty-five-year-old girl who died? That she was beautiful and brilliant. That she loved Mozart and Bach. The Beatles. And me."[11] Captured in the amber of literature, her death remains, in the narrator's voice, a sign that she cannot really die, any more than can Little Nell. Her memory captured in the text has made her perfection immortal. It is the memory of *The Virgin Suicides* that frame the 1993 debut novel by the American writer Jeffrey Eugenides. These young women cannot die any more than that other seemingly immortal Victorian character, Bram Stoker's *Dracula* (1897), whose eventual death is ever recycled in literature and the cinema. Dracula's body encased in a coffin filled with his native soil cannot decay but rather crumbles into dust when he is finally stabbed through the heart. Death, especially the beautiful, literary death, is in truth a denial of death; it is "the great boon of repression is that it makes it possible to live decisively in an overwhelmingly miraculous and incomprehensible world, a world so full of beauty, majesty, and terror that if animals perceived it all they would be paralyzed to act."[12] The dead body remains intact, whole, unblemished, indeed beautiful, rather than ugly, decayed, and corrupt. It is decay that is feared in life as well as in death. Indeed, Death's abstract body, the Grim Reaper, as Karl Rosenkranz notes in his *Aesthetics of Ugliness* (1853), is stripped of its decaying flesh and represented aesthetically as a skeleton with a scythe.[13] It becomes a Victorian icon.[14]

The body of the beautiful dying woman, the icon of a beautiful death, is always mourned: by her grandfather (and pet) in Dickens, by her lover in Dumas, Segal, and Eugenides. Someone is always left to acknowledge death, to serve as a surrogate for the mourner. Someone waiting for death but quite alive, like S. T. Coleridge's Ancient Mariner (1798), must tell the tale for those long dead and unable to do so. We can easily acknowledge, as John Bowen does in dismissing F. R. Leavis's indictment of Little Nell is nothing but "a contrived unreality" aiming to indulge in quenching the reader's thirst for sentimentalism, that the modern dislike of such deaths misses the literary point.[15] Little Nell is not a person, but an allegory. Her intentional "unreality" is an inherent aesthetic quality of her allegoric status rather than a lack. The question becomes an allegory for what?

Hebrews, Hellenes, Nazis

After 1933, daily life in Nazi Germany was all too full of the brutality of death. On the streets and in university lecture halls brown-shirted bullies beat and murdered Jews, Communists, and anyone else as they wished. Fleeing from the Nazis to Istanbul in 1935, the German-Jewish literary scholar Erich Auerbach examined what he understood to be the great divide between the Greeks and the Hebrews in their means of representing and therefore understanding the world, including death. To escape his own confrontation with death in the streets and his life in exile, textual aesthetics comes to capture his attention. The traditional dichotomy between Hebrews and Hellenes, between Jews and Greeks, as the embodiment of the antithesis of cultures haunted the nineteenth century, from G. W. F. Hegel to Heinrich Heine to Matthew Arnold. Jews and Greeks simply imagined the world differently, and this difference was embodied in their texts, especially in those representing death and dying. But this difference, more importantly, reflected for European culture the essential difference between the

Jews and the Greeks. This constructed difference enabled European thinkers to make a radical if arbitrary distinction between what they saw as the origin of European culture.

In Auerbach's *Mimesis* (eventually published in 1946), he comes to see Hellenistic textual representations of the world as embodied in Homer's depiction of Odysseus's scar as a "fully externalized description, uniform illustration, uninterrupted connection, free expression, all events in the foreground, displaying unmistakable meanings."[16] In other words, it is the detail of the world in which the Greeks lived that captured their attention, which accounts for everything from Homer to Aristotle, from literary device to atomic theory. The deaths in *The Iliad* also reflect this attention to detail. From the Trojan Agenor killing Elephenor by thrusting a spear in his side (4.543) to the Greek Achilles killing Hector, cutting through his throat without robbing him of the power of speech (22.410), and then mutilating his corpse by piercing his tendons of both feet behind from heel to ankle and by threading ox-hide thongs through them dragging him through the dust, Homeric deaths are detailed and precise.[17]

Homer's representation of death rests, as Auerbach quite correctly saw in his reading of the Greeks, on the details, on the finesse of the stroke, on the trailing, dusty hair. But it also represents a finality, a death that terminates life, concentrated in these details. Death for the Greeks is captured in the mourning rituals of the living: for instance, in Antigone's desperate need to bury the rotting corpse of her brother, Polynices. As Auerbach recognizes, it is details of this kind that make the text live for the reader.

Auerbach found the antithesis to this world of detail in *Genesis*. Here he actually presents a tale of death and dying as the prototype for the Hebrew means of representing death as a symbolic rather than as a realistic moment in the text. In the Akedah, the binding of Isaac,[18] he sees

> certain parts brought into high relief, others left obscure, abruptness, suggestive influence of the unexpressed, "background" quality, multiplicity of meanings and the need for interpretation, universal-historical claims, development of the concept of the historically becoming, and preoccupation with the problematic.[19]

Thus the Jews who, according to Auerbach following the "higher criticism" of the day, wrote the text and saw the world in exactly the opposite manner than the Greeks. Homer exemplifies the Greeks' tendency for realism; the Akedah, written with the skeletal and evocative nature of Jewish texts, demanding the necessary interpretation and reinterpretation so present in the millennia of readings of this central text. Death always demands explication in this context.

> And it came to pass after these things, that God did tempt Abraham, and said unto him, Abraham: and he said, Behold, here I am.
>
> And he said, Take now thy son, thine only son Isaac, whom thou lovest, and get thee into the land of Moriah; and offer him there for a burnt offering upon one of the mountains which I will tell thee of.
>
> . . . And Abraham took the wood of the burnt offering, and laid it upon Isaac his son; and he took the fire in his hand, and a knife; and they went both of them together.
>
> And Isaac spake unto Abraham his father, and said, My father: and he said, Here am I, my son. And he said, Behold the fire and the wood: but where is the lamb for a burnt offering?
>
> And Abraham said, My son, God will provide himself a lamb for a burnt offering: so they went both of them together.
>
> And they came to the place, which God had told him of; and Abraham built an altar there, and laid the wood in order, and bound Isaac his son, and laid him on the altar upon the wood.
>
> And Abraham stretched forth his hand, and took the knife to slay his son.
>
> And the angel of the Lord called unto him out of heaven, and said, Abraham, Abraham: and he said, Here am I.
>
> And he said, Lay not thine hand upon the lad, neither do thou any thing unto him: for now I know that thou fearest God, seeing thou hast not withheld thy son, thine only son from me.
>
> And Abraham lifted up his eyes, and looked, and behold behind him a ram caught in a thicket by his horns: and Abraham went and took the ram, and offered him up for a burnt offering in the stead of his son.

But wait: Unlike in *The Iliad* or in Sophocles's drama, in the tale of the binding of Abraham no one (except the ram) actually dies. Isn't the point that Abraham intends to sacrifice his son (Isaac if you follow the Judeo-Christian reading; Ishmael in the Quran 37:101–113) but *doesn't*? It is the slaughter of the accidental animal substitute, the scapegoat, that introduces death into the tale. Perhaps that symbolic substitute is the key to all of our Western readings of death in literature after all.

Christ and the Gift of Death

In *The Gift of Death,* Jacques Derrida notes that "narrative is genealogical but it is not simply an act of memory. It bears witness, in the manner of an ethical or political act, for today and for tomorrow. It means first of all thinking about what takes place today."[20] Every tale that is told and heard, every narrative we read or reread, is comprehended in terms of the ethical contradictions in our own world. There is no theme that better fits Derrida's formula concerning the collapse of a hierarchy of ethics in the modern world than narratives of sacrifice and dying. Modernity no longer has the comfort of the sort of transcendental hierarchy of sacrifice as found in Søren Kierkegaard. Kierkegaard, evoking the Akedah in his *Fear and Trembling* (1843), sees Abraham's refusal to strike as recognizing his unquestioned obligation to his innocent son transcending even divine command. In modernity, Derrida claims, an individual may have complex and contradictory affiliations and therefore be unable to "respond responsibly" to any given situation. Ambiguity and doubt result.

Derrida's account also grapples with our Biblical tale of the *Akedah,* Abraham's potential sacrifice of Isaac. He explores the aesthetic implications of our understanding of the creation of death stories that are in the end always life stories. The *Akedah,* for all of its complexity and contradictions, ends without a human death, but instead with a substitute sacrifice. In complex ways this very Jewish literary trope of the avoidance of human death (and the presence of sacrifice in all of its meanings nevertheless) is transformed into the core belief of all forms of Christianity, the actual death and physical resurrection of Jesus.

The authors of the Gospels sought to make a Jewish concept of death *without* death understandable to a growing and changing Gentile readership. There is, in contrast to Genesis, an emphasis on what René Girard calls "the sacrificial crisis," where Jesus becomes the focus of anxiety about the violence present in society itself—a violence between Roman and Jew, between Sadducees and Pharisees.[21] This violence is given a textual representation in the Gospels through a radical rereading of the Akedah. Death is not avoided by a substitute, but experienced by the very body of Christ, a surrogate for our own. His mortal body, captured at death in all its horror in Matthias Grünewald's altarpiece in the hospital chapel at Isenheim (1512–1516) that depicts the scarred and bloody body of the crucified Christ is transformed by the resurrection into the transfigured body of the Christ risen and ascending. The rotting, corrupt mortal body in death becomes the perfect and beautiful body of the divine.

Over the course of the four Gospels, the language articulated by the dying Jesus defines him as the sacrifice because he willingly gives up his corporeal being for his divine role: "For Christ also hath once suffered for sins, the just for the unjust, that he might bring us to God, being put to death in the flesh, but quickened by the Spirit."[22] At the very moment of his death, Jesus is reported by two of the Gospels to have cited Psalm 22:1 (David's cry, "My God, my God, why has Thou forsaken me? I cry in the daytime but Thou hearest not and the night-time and am not silent,"), not in Hebrew, but in Aramaic. In the first Gospel, Mark, Jesus "at the ninth hour . . . [cries] with a loud voice, saying 'Eloi, Eloi, Lama Sabachthani?'" which is, being interpreted, "My God, My God, why hast thou forsaken me?"[23] The onlookers in Mark mistakenly hear Jesus calling for Elijah rather than for God. But this is a cry of desperation, of the sacrifice of Jesus's corporal body without any promise of resurrection, it is a misunderstood message, as the listeners present misconstrue it. Matthew, written subsequently, alters Jesus's last words: "And about the ninth hour Jesus cried with a loud voice, saying, 'Eli, Eli, Lama Sabachthani?'" making the bystanders' misunderstanding still more plausible.[24] Jesus is here speaking the language of the Jews, of the "Old" Testament: his words are translated within the gospel text for readers to understand what he is saying, and to overcome the actual misunderstanding of the bystanders. In the later Gospel accounts of the passion, Christ speaks "directly" to the reader. In the parallel passage in Luke, Jesus is taken to Calvary and there is crucified. "And when Jesus had cried with a loud voice, he said, Father, into thy hands I commend my spirit: and having said thus, he gave up the ghost."[25] In John, the last of the Gospels that relates the life of Jesus, Christ is taken to Golgotha, and there "he said, It is finished: and he bowed his head, and gave up the ghost."[26] But of course it was not finished, as Luke and John intimate, and as the Nicene Creed states: "On the third day he rose again in accordance with the Scriptures." The sense of real death transformed is only present when the Gospels begin to address a universal readership rather than a Jewish one.

Modern Death between the Akedah and the Crucifixion

The sacrifice without human death in the Akedah is reflected into Christ's passion, death, and resurrection. Jewish commentators do not argue this. Whether the Akedah may be, as both Auerbach and the eleventh-century Iberian sage Yona Ibn Janach imply, symbolic of something much greater than themselves. Whether it may be a surrogate for all religious human beings, as Joseph B. Soloveitchik wrote: "The chosen of the nation, from the moment that they revealed God, occupied themselves in a continual act of sacrifice."[27] Lippman Bodoff sees Abraham and Isaac as representations of a real father who never would actually sacrifice his son, evidence for a God who could never truly demand such a thing.[28] J. H. Hertz argues that the account of Abraham and Isaac flies in the face of social conventions of Abraham's time about child sacrifice. Neither sees it as a textual prefiguration of death and resurrection; its textual presence resists a reading of actual death.[29] It is clear, as Sidra DeKoven Ezrahi observes, that

> as the Jews came to live more and more within the elastic bounds of their own internal discourse, the significant historical and geographic coordinates of collective life were located in the suspended time and place of sacred texts, and a lamentation tradition based on archetypal rather than historical memory evolved.[30]

It is the text itself that harbors immortality as well as mourning. "Et in Arcadia ego," says Death, but as Virgil shows in his memento mori in the *Eclogues*,[31] it is art in all its forms that seizes the moment of death and freezes it in a denial of death.

The Akedah becomes a central model for death and dying in the modern Western literary tradition only through its later transformation into the Christian model of death and resurrection. Do we believe that death can be avoided, or do we maintain that death is a necessity? Literary death sets this question aside while appearing to address it. Think about the body of Frankenstein's monster in Mary Shelley's novel of 1818. It is composed of fragments from dead bodies revitalized or resurrected through science. Yet his enormous form, his yellow skin and eyes mark him not as uncorrupted, a new Adam, but as the fallen angel that he calls himself. Yet Frankenstein's corrupt monster is revitalized over and over again in every reading, in every viewing, in every new version. Whether heralded or denied, this notion of a death denied through the act of reading is the lynchpin of literary deaths. And that includes the responses to Little Nell.

The Victorians as the Moderns

The Victorians were secular and Christian, in equal measure. They created secular nondenominational cemeteries such as Père Lachaise in 1804 in Paris, and Anglican, but inclusive, cemeteries such as Highgate in London in 1839. The Victorians were opposed to cremation, because it would deny the resurrection of the body. Yet a crematorium designed by Jean Camille Formigé opened in Père Lachaise in 1894, while Highgate still had none.[32] This tension was of the time. Victorian writers and their French contemporaries were fascinated by good deaths. There are eleven deaths in Emily Brontë's *Wuthering Heights* (1847), none more evocative than the dramatic deathbed scene of eighteen-year-old Catherine Earnshaw, who leaves her bed for a final rendezvous with Heathcliff. Catherine is dead before the novel begins, so that the narrator, knowing everything, remains the storehouse of memory transcending death. Catherine's death does not even terminate her life, at least in Heathcliff's fantasy. She continues to haunt him until his own death:

> He muttered detached words also; the only one I could catch was the name of Catherine, coupled with some wild term of endearment or suffering; and spoken as one would speak to a person present; low and earnest, and wrung from the depth of his soul.[33]

In Charlotte Brontë's *Jane Eyre* (1847), the angelic consumptive Helen Burns is called to heaven from Lowood School, where she refused to hate those who abused her and never lost her faith in God:

> We are, and must be, one and all, burdened with faults in this world: but the time will soon come when, I trust, we shall put them off in putting off our corruptible bodies; when debasement and sin will fall from us with this cumbrous frame of flesh, and only the spark of the spirit will remain,—the impalpable principle of light and thought, pure as when it left the Creator to inspire the creature: whence it came it will return; perhaps again to be communicated to some being higher than man—perhaps to pass through gradations of glory, from the pale human soul to brighten to the seraph![34]

No pretense of secularization here. The promise of freedom from death in the Christian tradition is made explicit in the text.

But what about Little Nell and *The Old Curiosity Shop*? Her grandfather survives her, mad, seated at her grave until "they laid him by the side of her whom he had loved so well; and, in the church where they had often prayed and mused, and lingered hand in hand, the child and the old man slept together."[35] Unlike the ram in Genesis, the pet bird does survive. (Dickens borrows these figures—from the anonymous aged and mad Harper and the beautiful and duteous, Mignon, too soon dead—directly from Goethe's *Wilhelm Meister Apprenticeship* [1795–6] in Thomas Carlyle's 1824 translation.) Life after death? A faith that is affirmed? Dickens asserts after Nell's death that

> it is not on earth that Heaven's justice ends. Think what it is, compared with the World to which her young spirit has winged its early flight; and say, if one deliberate wish expressed in solemn terms above this bed could call her back to life, which of us would utter it![36]

But the true end lies with the narrator after all of the deaths above: "The magic reel, which, rolling on before, has led the chronicler thus far, now slackens in its pace, and stops. It lies before the goal; the pursuit is at an end."[37] Only the Olympian narrator is immortal, beyond death. The book may end, but it remains a living thing, ever brought to life by new readers and readings.

The Akedah presents the promise of resolution, but like the ironic responses of the moderns to Little Nell's death, it too becomes mired in a skepticism driven by readers' experiences of death. Oscar Wilde's comment on Little Nell's death evoking laughter can only be understood in the light of his anxiety about the promise of resurrection, mirrored in the eternal youth and damnation of Dorian Gray (1890):

> Ah! in what a monstrous moment of pride and passion he had prayed that the portrait should bear the burden of his days, and he keep the unsullied splendour of eternal youth! All his failure had been due to that. Better for him that each sin of his life had brought its sure swift penalty along with it. There was purification in punishment. Not "Forgive us our sins" but "Smite us for our iniquities" should be the prayer of man to a most just God.[38]

Dorian Gray became one of the bits of evidence brought against Wilde during his trials for sodomy, but one could also imagine here a prefiguration of his deathbed conversion to Roman Catholicism and his posthumous resurrection as a gay saint.

Modern Life and Death in WWI

By 1918, well after Wilde's death in Paris in 1900, the theme of death seemed best captured by a modernist reading of the denial of death. Would such a divine father have really sacrificed his sons? As the

WWI British poet Wilfred Owen implies in his extraordinary poem on the Akedah, "The Parable Of The Old Man And The Young" (1918):

> So Abram rose, and clave the wood, and went,
> And took the fire with him, and a knife.
> And as they sojourned both of them together,
> Isaac the first-born spake and said, My Father,
> Behold the preparations, fire and iron,
> But where the lamb for this burnt-offering?
> Then Abram bound the youth with belts and straps,
> and builded parapets and trenches there,
> And stretchèd forth the knife to slay his son.
> When lo! an angel called him out of heaven,
> Saying, Lay not thy hand upon the lad,
> Neither do anything to him. Behold,
> A ram, caught in a thicket by its horns;
> Offer the Ram of Pride instead of him. But the old man would not so, but slew his son,
> And half the seed of Europe, one by one.[39]

No possible staying of the hand; no resurrection. This becomes part of the vocabulary of aesthetic modernism through mid-century, exemplified in the fourteen black-and-white minimalist paintings that make up the entirety of Barnett Newman's post-Holocaust series entitled *Stations of the Cross* (1958–66). Their subtitle is Christ's lament: "lema lema sabachthani." The American Jewish painter understands this lament not only as the first portion of Psalm 22 but also as the introduction of a universal and radical interpenetration and disruption of any clarity or distinction between Christ as Christian Messiah and Jesus as a suffering Jew. The canvases in their minimalist aesthetic create a purity of form and vision that avoids any representation of the body, defiled or resurrected.

Franz Kafka, writing at virtually the same moment as Wilfred Owen, sees the Akedah not as a denial of death but as an affirmation of its finality. No text is clearer in this regard than "A Fratricide" (1919).[40] In this tale, "Schmar, the murderer" whets "his weapon, half a bayonet and half a kitchen knife" on his boot while he waits for his victim, Wese. Schmar slaughters Wese: "And right into the throat and left into the throat and a third time deep into the belly stabbed Schmar's knife."[41] This ritual reenactment of the Akedah is heightened by Schmar's shriek: "The bliss of murder! The relief, the soaring ecstasy from the shedding of another's blood! Wese, old night bird, friend, alehouse crony, you are oozing away into the dark earth below the street. Why aren't you simply a bladder of blood so that I could stamp on you and make you vanish into nothingness?"[42] His victim is not merely a "bladder of blood" but a living, breathing individual whose murder is ritualized, but in the end the murder is apprehended by the policeman. Order is restored, at least superficially. This text echoes the final scene in *The Trial* (1914), where K. is taken out and executed:

> The two of them laid K. down on the ground, propped him up against the boulder, and settled his head upon it. But in spite of the pains they took and all the willingness K. showed, his posture remained contorted and unnatural-looking. . . . Then one of them opened his frock coat and out of a sheath that hung from a belt girt round his waistcoat drew a long, thin, double-edged butcher's knife, held it up, and tested the cutting edges in the moonlight. . . . [K.] raised his hands and spread out all his fingers.
>
> But the hands of one of the partners were already at K.'s throat, while the other thrust the knife deep into his heart and turned it twice. With failing eyes K. could still see the two of them immediately before him, cheek leaning against cheek, watching the final act. "Like a dog!" he said; it was as if the shame of it must outlive him.[43]

The ritual is a parody of the Akedah. Here it is the opening of the body, the stab into the heart, that reveals the awful truth about what one has really been all along. K.'s last thought is that he is being murdered like an unclean animal, a dog, rather than like a ritually pure one, such as a ram. His thought recalls the dog from Kafka's tale of "Jackals and Arabs," first published in Martin Buber's periodical *The Jew* in October 1917, where it is the jackals whose uncleanness is a reflection of the world's attitude toward the Jews. The jackals plan a murder of the Arabs. What must be done, says one old jackal, is that "we shall draw blood from them, and the quarrel will be over."[44] It is the drawing of blood that will cure. But they are too cowardly and weak to draw this blood themselves: "And so, sir," they say to the European visitor, "and so, dear sir, by means of your all-powerful hands slit their throats through with these scissors!" The tool provided for their execution is a "small pair of sewing scissors, covered with ancient rust."

Kafka's representation of the crucified body, if there is one in his published literary work, is to be found in the scene of impalement of the officer at the close of "In the Penal Colony" (1919). The "remarkable piece of apparatus" designed by the "Old Commandant" on Kafka's version of Devil's Island had been designed repeatedly to inscribe the crime on the prone body of a condemned man until he is transfigured with an awareness of his crime. At the close of the tale the machine collapses on the body of the executioner as it:

> was not writing but only jabbing, and the Bed was not turning the body over but only bringing it up quivering against the needles.... [T]his was no exquisite torture such as the officer desired; this was plain murder.... And now the last action failed to fulfill itself, the body did not drop off the long needles, streaming with blood it went on hanging over the pit without falling into it.... [H]e had to look at the face of the corpse. It was as it had been in life; no sign was visible of the promised redemption; what the others had found in the machine, the officer had not found; the lips were firmly pressed together, the eyes were open, with the same expression as in life, his look was calm and convinced, through the forehead went the point of the great iron spike.[45]

The machine disfigures the corpse rather than transfiguring it. It is a slaughtering of the body as certainly as the soldiers' bodies were butchered in the trenches. Kafka's literary bodies are mutilated. In his dreams Kafka feels himself mutilated by the "pork butcher's broad knife that quickly and with mechanical regularity chops into me from the side and cuts off very thin slices that fly off almost like shavings because of the speed of the action."[46] The executed officer as well as K. become essential victims, robbed of their integrity and manliness, murdered ritually by the world about them.

The rejection of a denial of death after WWI becomes almost commonplace. In Thomas Mann's *The Magic Mountain* (1924), the figure of Leo Naphta, whom the protagonist Hans Castorp meets in the tuberculosis sanitarium at Davos, is immediately revealed to the reader as a Jew by his "corrosive ugliness":

> Everything about him was sharp: the hooked nose dominating his face, the narrow, pursed mouth, the thick, beveled lenses of his glasses in their light frame, behind which were a pair of pale-gray eyes—even the silence he preserved, which suggested that when he broke it, his speech would be incisive and logical.[47]

Naphta's Jewish background opens the novel to an understanding of death and sacrifice that is an ironic counterpoint to the sanatorium. Leo (or as he was then called, Leib) Naphta came from the Eastern reaches of the Austrian Empire, from the Galician-Volhynian border, where his father Elie was a ritual slaughterer:

> Standing near the victim, which was hobbled and bound indeed, but not stunned, he would lift the mighty slaughter-knife and bring it to rest in a deep gash close to the cervical vertebra; while the assistant held the quickly filling basins to receive the gushing, steaming blood, and the child looked on the sight with that childish gaze that often pierces through the sense into the essential, and may have been in an unusual degree the gift of the starry-eyed Elie's son. He knew that Christian butchers had to stun their cattle with a blow from a club before killing them, and that this regulation was made in order to avoid unnecessary cruelty. Yet his father, so fine and so intelligent by comparison with those louts, and starry-eyed as never one of them, did his task according to the Law, striking down the creature while its senses were undimmed, and letting its life-blood well out until it sank. The boy Leib felt that the stupid *goyim* were actuated by an easy and irreverent good nature, which paid less honor to the deity that did his father's solemn mercilessness; thus the conception of piety came to be bound up in his mind with that of cruelty, and the idea of the sacred and the spiritual with the sight and smell of spurting blood.[48]

While his is a somewhat standard representation of Jewish ritual slaughter, it also immediately evokes the Akedah, the animal scapegoat sacrificed to allow man to live. Mann, never one to leave well enough alone, lays out the mythic continuum on which Naphta's spiritual type must be placed. For Elie Naphta is also a "familiar of God, a Baal-Shem or Zaddik, a miracle man" who can cure "a woman of a malignant sore, and another time a boy of spasms, simply by means of blood and invocations." Mann continues this line of associations, for in the very next sentences, he describes Elie Naphta's eventual fate:

> But it was precisely this aura of an uncanny piety, in which the odor of his blood-bolstered calling played a part, that proved his destruction. There had been the unexplained death of two gentile boys, a popular uprising, a panic of rage—and Elie had died horribly, nailed crucifix-wise on the door of his burning home.

No death without death but a crucifixion, the ultimate sacrifice but here in this secular world of death without the possibility of resurrection.

Leo Naptha is at Davos being treated for tuberculosis because his mother was tubercular. According to Mann, Leo has "the seeds of his lung disease" from his mother and from his father "beside his slenderness of build, an extraordinary intelligence." Naptha is the regressive pedagogical force (opposed to Septtembrini and Peeperkorn) in the fictive world of Mann's "magic mountain." But the only truly modern figure in the novel remains the protagonist Hans Castorp, who learns from experience, under the motto *placet experiri,* rather than from books or tradition—and who is not actually tubercular! For him it is the vicarious experience of death and dying in the sanatorium that serves as his introduction to life, much like the Tower Society in Goethe's *Wilhelm Meister's Apprenticeship* is his means of learning about the world beyond. It is the Akedah now made secular with Davos as the new Mount Moriah.

Freud's Little Walk

Death in fiction, even Little Nell's, is never final, because—and this is the truth that binds all—the reader always lives, is always renewed, is always resurgent. Death waits for us in fiction. Sigmund Freud, hiking in the Dolomites "in the summer before the war," presents his high Victorian (or perhaps better: Imperial Austrian) view, that of one of his favorite authors, Charles Dickens, in a debate with two much younger compatriots[49]:

> Transience value is scarcity value in time. Limitation in the possibility of an enjoyment raises the value of the enjoyment. It was incomprehensible, I declared, that the thought of the transience of beauty should interfere with our joy in it. . . . The beauty of the human form and face vanish forever in the course of our own lives, but their evanescence only lends them a fresh charm. A time may indeed come when the pictures and statues which we admire to-day will crumble to dust, or a race of men may follow us who no longer understand the works of our poets and thinkers, or a geological epoch may even arrive when all animate life upon the earth ceases; but since the value of all this beauty and perfection is determined only by its significance for our own emotional lives, it has no need to survive us and is therefore independent of absolute duration.

But the "young but already famous poet" (Rainer Maria Rilke, perhaps) and the friend (Lou Andreas Salome?) who accompanies him cannot agree with this sense of inevitable bodily decay and the role of beauty as a means emotionally to escape such a confrontation. They, living at the moment when death is not beautiful, but ambivalent, counter his argument:

> These considerations appeared to me incontestable; but I noticed that I had made no impression either upon the poet or upon my friend. My failure led me to infer that some powerful emotional factor was

> at work, which was disturbing their judgment, and I believed later that I had discovered what it was. What spoilt their enjoyment of beauty must have been a revolt in their minds against mourning. The idea that all this beauty was transient was giving these two sensitive minds a foretaste of mourning over its decease; and, since the mind instinctively recoils from anything that is painful, they felt their enjoyment of beauty interfered with by thoughts of its transience.[50]

For the young at the turn of the twentieth century beauty evokes transience, evokes death, evokes loss. But it is melancholy for an object not quite real to us, the fictive object of death; not mourning, with our relationship to real memories of real individuals, but the melancholic, repetitive evocation of death as it is in reading: never altered, always constant. As Freud noted, this sense antedated the Great War for "a year later the war broke out and robbed the world of its beauties. . . . It robbed us of very much that we had loved, and showed us how ephemeral were many things that we had regarded as changeless."[51] The quotidian dead, the bodies in the trenches are now too real, too corrupted not to draw into question what had been a truth about beauty and death. We, still immured in modernity, remember not death, but instead see its shadow in the death of Little Nell. Hers is an unreal death, a death with the promise of resurrection, a promise undermined on later rereading by modernity's anxiety about that promise.

In fiction we vacillate between admiring the beauty of death, a beauty that signifies its vanquishing, and a fascination with our mourning about death, vicariously experienced, that mirrors our sense of loss. J. K. Rowling knows that full well when she builds her *The Casual Vacancy* (2012) on the sudden death of the forty-four-year-old Barry Fairbrother, *nomen est omen*, in the opening chapter, triggering the entire flow of the novel. The novel culminates in a double death of children—not the beautiful, gracious children of Dickens. They are Krystal and Robbie Weedon, the abused and abandoned children of The Fields. The name of their home is a contemporary British irony that converts the newly constructed and unwanted slums for the "undeserving poor" into the Elysium Fields. This is a novel about death as both the product of modernity and as a moment of accidental betrayal. Rowling's highly modern sense is that death is horrid but that it can redeem: after all of the chaos following the initial sudden death and the horrors of the children's deaths at the close of the novel, death causes transformation. The death is not transformative in the Victorian sense. As Rowling ironically observes, the drowned three-year-old Robbie Weedon is transformed by the gossips of the town into a modern Little Nell: "The dirty and foul-mouthed little boy, of whose existence few had been aware . . . was spoken of everywhere as a water baby, a cherub, a pure and gentle angel whom all would have embraced with love and compassion, if only they could have saved him."[52] But at least one of the characters, the self-harming, self-hating teen Sukhvinder Jawanda, is transformed by these deaths into an aware and self-confident young adult. Death redeems, it rescues, if it is a death without death, a life-affirming death, for which all readers await—the death in fiction, a thought experiment perhaps first undertaken by God in Genesis.[53]

Notes

1. All references are to Charles Dickens, *The Old Curiosity Shop*, ed. Elizabeth M. Brennan (Oxford: Oxford University Press, 1997), here 557. See also Marilyn Georgas, "Little Nell and the Art of Holy Dying: Dickens and Jeremy Taylor," *Dickens Studies Annual: Essays on Victorian Fiction* 20 (1991): 35–56; Jolene Zigarovich, *Writing Death and Absence in the Victorian Novel: Engraved Narratives* (New York: Palgrave Macmillan, 2012).
2. Linda and Michael Hutcheon, *Opera: Desire, Disease, Death* (Lincoln: University of Nebraska Press, 1996) and *Opera: The Art of Dying* (Cambridge, MA: Harvard University Press, 2004).
3. Karl S. Guthke, *The Gender of Death: A Cultural History in Art and Literature* (Cambridge: Cambridge University Press, 1999) and Elisabeth Bronfen, *Over Her Dead Body: Death, Femininity, and the Aesthetic* (Manchester: Manchester University Press, 2006).
4. Seneca, *Four Tragedies and Octavia*, trans. E. F. Watling (Harmondsworth: Penguin, 2005), 129.
5. Rainer Maria Rilke, *The Notebooks Of Malte Laurids Brigge*, trans. Stephen Mitchell (New York: Random House, 1982), 43.
6. Queen Victoria's Journals, Entry for 5 March 1841. Last modified 2012. http://www.queenvictoriasjournals.org/ (accessed December 6th, 2013).
7. Laurence Lerner, *Angels and Absences: Child Deaths in the 19th Century* (Nashville, TN: Vanderbilt University Press, 1997), 180.
8. Algernon Charles Swinburne, "The Greatness of Dickens," *The Bookman*. Extra Number: Charles Dickens, 183. (1914), 83–4.
9. Joseph Jacobs, "The Dying of Death," *Fortnightly Review* (August 1899): 264–69, here 264.
10. Aldous Huxley, *Vulgarity in Literature* (London: Chatto and Windus, 1930), 6.
11. Erich Segal, *Love Story* (New York: Harper and Row, 1970), 3.
12. Ernest Becker, *The Denial of Death* (New York: Simon & Schuster, 1973), 59.
13. Karl Rosenkranz, *Aesthetik des Hässlichen* (Königsberg: Gebrüder Bornträger, 1853), 315.
14. Ernest Becker, *The Denial of Death* (New York: Simon & Schuster, 1973), 59.
15. John Bowen, *Dickens and the Children of Empire* (New York: Palgrave Publishers, 2000), 14.

16. Erich Auerbach, *Mimesis: The Representation of Reality in Western Literature* (Garden City: Doubleday, 1957), 19.
17. Wolf-Hartmut Friedrich, *Wounding and Death in the Iliad: Homeric Techniques of Description*, trans. Gabriele Wright and Peter Jones (London: Duckworth, 2003).
18. Genesis 18:1–22:24
19. Auerbach, *Mimesis*, 23.
20. Jacques Derrida, *The Gift of Death*, trans. David Wills (Chicago: The University of Chicago Press), 35.
21. See René Girard, *Things Hidden Since the Foundation of the World* (Stanford, CA: Stanford University Press, 1987). Major texts that use Girard's theory to examine violence in religion are James Alison, *Raising Abel: The Recovery of Eschatological Imagination* (New York: Crossroads, 1996); Gil Bailie, *Violence Unveiled: Humanity at the Crossroads* (New York: Crossroad, 1995); and Walter Wink, *Engaging the Powers: Discernment and Resistance in a World of Domination* (Minneapolis: Fortress, 1992).
22. 1 Peter 18.
23. 15: 34.
24. 27: 46.
25. 23: 46.
26. 19: 30.
27. Joseph B. Soloveitchik, *Divrei Hashkafa*, ed. Moshe Krone (Jerusalem: World Zionist Organization, 1992), 255.
28. Lippman Bodoff, *The Binding of Isaac, Religious Murders & Kabbalah: Seeds of Jewish Extremism and Alienation?* (New York: Devora Publishing, 2005).
29. J. H. Hertz, *The Pentateuch and Haftorahs*, 5 vols. (London: Soncino Press, 1930–1936), 1: 229.
30. Sidra DeKoven Ezrahi, "Considering the Apocalypse: Is the Writing on the Wall Only Grafitti?" in Berel Lang, ed., *Writing and the Holocaust* (New York: Holmes and Meier, 1988), 137–159, here. 138–139.
31. V, 42.
32. Jonathan Strauss, *Human Remains: Medicine, Death, and Desire in Nineteenth-Century Paris* (New York; Fordham University Press, 2012).
33. Emily Bronte, *Wuthering Heights*, ed. Ian Jack (Oxford: Oxford University Press, 1999), 348.
34. Charlotte Bronte, *Jane Eyre*, ed., Michael Mason (New York: Penguin Books, 1996), 210–11.
35. Dickens, *Old Curiosity Shop*, 566.
36. Ibid., 558–9.
37. Ibid., 566.
38. Russell Jackson, Joseph Bristow, eds., *The Complete Works of Oscar Wilde: Vol. 3: The Picture of Dorian Gray* (Oxford: Oxford University Press, 2005), 354.
39. Wilfred Owen, "The Parable of the Old Man and the Young," *The Complete Poems and Fragments*, ed., Jon Stallworthy. *Volume I: The Poems* (London: Chatto & Windus / The Hogarth Press / Oxford University Press, 1983), 151. Wyatt Bonikowski, *Shell Shock and the Modernist Imagination: The Death Drive in Post–World War I British Fiction* (Farnham, England: Ashgate, 2013).

40. Franz Kafka, *The Complete Stories*, ed. Nahum N. Glatzer (New York: Schocken, 1971), 402–4. See Günter Blamberger, "Kafka's Death Images," in Bernhard Debatin, et al., ed., *Metaphor and Rational Discourse* (Tübingen: Niemeyer; 1997), 239–50.
41. Ibid., 403.
42. Ibid., 403.
43. Franz Kafka, *The Trial*, trans. Breon Mitchell (New York: Schocken, 1998), 227–9.
44. Kafka, *Stories*, 410.
45. Kafka, *Stories*, 165–66.
46. Franz Kafka, *The Trial*, op. cit., 227–9.
47. All references are to Thomas Mann, *The Magic Mountain*, trans. H. T. Lowe-Porter (New York: Alfred Knopf, 1982 [1924]), here 440–41. See Caroline Joan S. Picart, *Thomas Mann and Friedrich Nietzsche: Eroticism, Death, Music, and Laughter* (Amsterdam, Netherlands: Rodopi, 1999).
48. Mann, *Magic Mountain*, 440–441.
49. Hannah S. Decker, *Freud, Dora, and Vienna 1900* (New York: The Free Press, 1991), 133.
50. Sigmund Freud, "On Transience" [1916] in Sigmund Freud, *Standard Edition of the Complete Psychological Works of Sigmund Freud*, ed. and trans. J. Strachey, A. Freud, A. Strachey, and A. Tyson. 24 vols. (London: Hogarth, 1955–74), here 14: 304–5. Freud continues this argument in more detail in his essay on "Mourning and Melancholy" (1917). In reality Freud earlier met in Munch in the summer of 1913 with Rilke and Andreas Salome. See Matthew von Unwerth, *Freud's Requiem: Mourning, Memory and the Invisible History of a Summer Walk* (New York: Continuum 2006).
51. Freud, *Transience*, 306.
52. J. K. Rowling, *The Casual Vacancy* (New York: Little, Brown and Co., 2012), 485.
53. For further reading see: Philippa Berry, *Shakespeare's Feminine Endings: Disfiguring Death in the Tragedies* (London: Routledge, 1999); Douglas Davies, *A Brief History of Death* (Oxford: Blackwell, 2005); Carolyn Dever, *Death and the Mother from Dickens to Freud: Victorian Fiction and the Anxiety of Origins* (Cambridge: Cambridge University Press, 1998); Alan Warren Friedman, *Fictional Death and the Modernist Enterprise* (Cambridge; New York: Cambridge University Press, 1995); Paul Koudounaris, *The Empire of Death: A Cultural History of Ossuaries and Charnel Houses* (London: Thames & Hudson, 2011); Finnur Magnússon, "Narratives of Modern Dying: Looking for Authentic Death," *Pro Ethnologia* 4 (1996): 81–88; Sarah Mei-Wen Liu, "As We Lay Dying: Coming to Terms with Death in Literary Modernism," (PhD diss. University of California, Berkeley, 2000); Esther Schor, *Bearing The Dead: The British Culture of Mourning from the Enlightenment to Victoria* (Princeton, NJ: Princeton University Press, 1994); Richard Sugg, *Murder after Death: Literature and Anatomy in Early Modern England* (Ithaca, NY: Cornell University Press, 2007); Christiane Sourvinou-Inwood, *'Reading' Greek Death: To The End Of The Classical Period* (Oxford: Clarendon Press, 1995); Ruth Richardson, *Death, Dissection and the Destitute* (London and New York: Routledge and Kegan Paul, 1987).

Questions

Who defines "death"?

What are the medical definitions of death in the course of the twentieth century?

How is a medical definition of death different from a cultural definition of death?

Are there different religious definitions of death?

What is a "good" death"?

How does the sacrifice of Isaac serve as a model for a "death without death"?

How does the crucifixion serve as a model for Western understanding of death?

How can the representation of death in a literary work serve as a key to the cultural assumptions about death in a specific culture at a specific time?

Index

For Product Safety Concerns and Information please contact our EU representative GPSR@taylorandfrancis.com
Taylor & Francis Verlag GmbH, Kaufingerstraße 24, 80331 München, Germany

www.ingramcontent.com/pod-product-compliance
Ingram Content Group UK Ltd.
Pitfield, Milton Keynes, MK11 3LW, UK
UKHW022002180926
475701UK00003B/149

9781138510791